Magnetic Field Therapy

Bringing Harmony and Balance to Your Body

By R. Allen Walls

INNER SEARCH FOUNDATION, INC.
MCLEAN, VIRGINIA

Published by:

Inner Search Foundation, Inc.
P.O. Box 10382
McLean, VA 22102-1502

Magnetic Field Therapy Handbook, First Edition, Copyright 1993 by Inner Search Foundation, Inc.

Library of Congress Cataloging-in-Publication Data
Walls, Robert Allen (1941)
Magnetic Field Therapy Handbook
1. Magnetism and Energy -
Therapeutic Use
Bibliography
ISBN - 0-9621790-3-5

Other Books by the Author
Life Plan: Finding Your Real Self
(ISBN #0-9-621790-1-9)

We must act as though we were the masters of our destiny, as though all things were bound to obey us; and yet in our soul resides the true knowing to give over in noble submission to the mighty spiritual forces we will inevitably encounter.

Maurice Maeterlinck
Wisdom & Destiny—1903

The purpose of this handbook is to help you learn how to improve and maintain your health by using Magnetic Field Therapy to relieve stress and physical discomfort and to balance the overall energy field of your body.

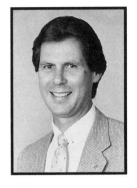

In my work as a therapist I use a total approach to wellness to help my clients achieve a positive spiritual, mental and physical condition.

The body is affected by all of the various conditions it is exposed to daily. Keeping the physical body in harmony and in proper balance is crucial. How well your body functions is dependent upon a complex interaction among the food you eat, everything you ingest or inhale (which could include addictive drugs, smoke, and harmful amounts of other substances), negative or positive environmental conditions, the amount of exercise you get, the amount of stress in your life, the atmosphere of love within and around you, and your connectedness with the positive forces in the universe.

Using Magnetic Field Therapy is a step toward taking command of your well-being and can lead you to an increased awareness of the value and importance of self care. It opens a new way for self examination. Explore all the areas of your body and feel how your energy field reacts to the use of Magnetic Field Therapy. The effect may be dramatic or may occur subtly over a period of time. Whichever effect occurs, you will be improving your health.

Happy days, a full and pleasurable life, can be yours whenever you are ready to put your spiritual, physical and mental health at the top of your list.

Take responsibility for your total well-being. Start NOW!

R. Allen Walls

About the Author

R. Allen Walls is a behavioral and core-energetic therapist. He is President of Inner Search Foundation, Inc., an educational and spiritual-development, non-profit, tax-exempt organization. Mr. Walls is the author of the book, *Life Plan, Finding Your Real Self, The Journey Through Life.* For more than fifteen years as a therapist, he has stressed the value of practicing a comprehensive approach to wellness along with developing a positive spiritual consciousness. He helps his clients connect with their higher purpose and attain an overall sense of well-being.

Dedication and Acknowledgments

This book is for my wife, Mari, who has helped me in every way with her loving support and encouragement, and for my children, Justin and Farrah, who have used Magnetic Field Therapy and support my healing work.

My thanks and appreciation to the following persons who have contributed immeasurably to the production of the book: Luella Murri for her dedication in editing the book with careful attention to the many details; Mary Anne Díaz, who made the graphics and typography so completely readable and understandable; and Al Crook for his original idea and for allowing this publication to become a reality.

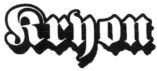

Kryon

In the past several years, Kryon, as named in the series of three books written by Lee Carroll, explained and presented messages from the spiritual realm.

Kryon is of Magnetic Service. Described as an entity of service, Kryon has never been a human or anything other than a spiritual form of magnetic service.

Which brings me to the reason for alerting you, the person who is interested in magnetic field application, to finding out more about the spiritual aspects of magnetic fields.

In the first Kryon book, Lee writes the message about how "We are all linked together." We are the great "I AM" as your Scriptures call God. When I send the message, "I am Kryon" there is a communication that I belong to the whole, and my signature is KRYON. We are GOD. You are a piece of GOD, and you have the power to become as high on your side of the veil as you were before you came... and you are loved without measure. You are each high entities of your own who have agreed to be exactly where you are before you ever got where you are. We are all collective in spirit, even while you are earth, veiled from truth."

I am recommending you begin to go deeper in your knowledge and learn the real importance about magnetic fields. Use the Kryon books series I, II, and III as a valuable part of your own learning and knowing.

You can contact Mr. Lee Carroll if you need help finding these books and want more information. In any event, I urge you to read them and gain much deeper awareness about your task on this planet.

For Contact with KRYON
Mr. Lee Carroll
The KRYON Writings
1155 Camino Del Mar, #422
Del Mar, California 92014   1-800-352-6657

Published by:

Inner Search Foundation, Inc.
P.O. Box 10382
McLean, VA 22102-1502

Magnetic Field Application Handbook, First Edition, Copyright 1993 by Inner Search Foundation, Inc.

Library of Congress Cataloging-in-Publication Data
Walls, R. Allen 1941
Magnetic Field Application Handbook
1. Magnetism and Energy - Therapeutic Use
Bibliography: P 1. Includes index
ISBN - 0-9621790-3-5

This Magnetic Field Application handbook is a publication of Inner Search Foundation, Inc., a non-profit 501(C), (3) tax-exempt organization. To order copies of this publication contact Inner Search Foundation, Inc., 1-703-448-3362.

Table of Contents

Introduction

Magnetic Field Therapy   5
How Magnetic Fields Affect the Body   7
    (From "An Overview of Biomagnetic Therapeutics"
    by Edward A. Hacmac, D.C.)
The Healing Crisis   10

Section 1 — Magnetic Field Therapy — Acupressure
        Method

Procedures   12
Cautions and Proper Usage   12
Problem Areas or Conditions and Applicable Procedures 14
    Greeting   17
    Metabolism   18
    Abdomen   19
    Back   20
    Ears   21
    Eyes   22
    Head   23
    Heart, Veins, Blood Pressure, Circulation   24
    Infection, Influenza, Allergy   25
    Lungs   26
    Neck   27
    Psoriasis, Stress, Shingles, Anxiety   28
    Shoulder   29
    Sinus   30
    Solar Plexus   31

Section 2 — Magnetic Field Therapy — Short and Long-Term Application

Flexible Magnetic Therapy Pads   32
Use of Flexible Magnetic Therapy Pads   33
Cautions and Proper Usage   33
Suggestions for Short- and Long-Term Application
    of Magnetic Field Therapy   35

    Ankle   35
    Arthritis   35
    Asthma   36
    Back (High & Low)   36
    Bags Under the Eyes   37
    Carpal Tunnel Syndrome   38
    Feet   38
    Hand Joints   39
    Hips   40
    Knees   40
    Menstrual Cramps   41
    Neck   41
    Phantom Limb Pain   41
    Shoulder Pain   42
    Sinus Headaches   42
    Stress Headaches   43
    Temporal Mandibular Joint   43
    Tennis, Racquet Ball or Squash Elbow   44
    Thumb   44
    Wrinkles on the Face   45
    Wrist Strains   45

Magnetic Field Therapy for Total Body Wellness   46

Magnetized Drinking Water—   48
    Cleansing Your Body Internally

Section 3 — Articles and Excerpts concerning Magnetic Field Therapy

Revolutionary New Magnetic Therapy KO's 49
    Arthritis Pain, by Jim O'Brien, *Your Health*,
    April 6, 1993

A Summary of Beneficial Influence of Magnetic Therapy, 54
    from *Magnetic Therapy*, by Dr. H. L. Bansal

New Applications for the Treatment of Pain, 56
    Fatigue, and Sleep Disorders, by Robert Lang, M.D.

Magnetism - The Force That's Always With You, 59
    by Curt Suplee, *The Washington Post*,
    page H1, December 14, 1994

Magnetic Field Therapy: Professional 63
and Personal Observations by Edward Friedler, M.D.

Magnetic Field Therapy: A Doctor's Experience, 66
    by William W. Lampard, M.D.

Why Magnetic Therapy Works, by Leane E. Roffey 70

Suggestions for Application of Biomagnetic 83
    Therapy Devices for Equine Use

An Overview of Biomagnetic Therapeutics, 87
    by Edward A. Hacmac, D.C.

Clinical Test of Magnetic Mattresspads, 99
    by Dr. Kazuo Shimodaira

References 101

Ordering Information 103

Human beings evolved and live within the earth's magnetic field, which is essential to the life of every living cell. However, scientific measurements show that the strength of the magnetic field has decreased over the centuries. Furthermore, animals die if shielded from the earth's magnetic force. Whereas during most of our evolutionary history we spent much or all of our time outdoors, many of us now spend a large part of every day in buildings which block the earth's magnetic field.

Dr. Robert O. Becker, pioneering researcher and author of the books, *The Body Electric* and *Cross Currents*, has established that the energy system within our bodies consists of two forces, magnetism and electricity, with the electricity component consisting of a low-frequency direct-current (DC) electric field. This electromagnetic energy system is affected by the earth's natural electromagnetic environment, which is normally relatively quiet, with minor rhythmic variations, but which experiences wild fluctuations and great increases in strength during magnetic storms. Our bodies resonate to the rhythm of earth's normally quiet field and are disturbed by marked changes in that field.

Today the earth is being blanketed with abnormal man-made electromagnetic fields produced by alternating currents (AC) in a wide range of frequencies, by radio waves, and by microwaves. Sources include electrical and electronic appliances in home and workplace, computers, high-voltage power lines, and world-wide communications systems. Dr. Becker calls this condition "electropollution." He states that it interferes with the earth's natural electromagnetic field and that it has been shown to have serious biological effects on living organisms. Other researchers warning of the harmful effects of "electric smog" have included the U.S. Surgeon General.

Magnetic Field Therapy products have now been designed especially to provide the natural magnetism needed for total body wellness, as well as to subtly stimulate the body's own healing mechanism in the case of stress and specific physical problems.

The recommended products are those with a strength of fewer than 1,000 Gauss, since magnets with a higher strength should be used only under professional supervision. The magnets are permanent and can be used indefinitely without losing their strength.

This *Magnetic Field Therapy Handbook* has been prepared to help people who seek overall well-being, as well as those who suffer from stress and specific physical problems.

The handbook describes two different ways to use specially designed flexible magnetic therapy pads. The pattern of alternating triangles of north and south poles makes these pads more effective than ordinary magnets.

Section One describes the Acupressure Method, in which magnetic therapy pads are held briefly on specific points along the acupressure meridians (energy channels) to increase and balance the flow of energy through the body. The placement of the magnets corresponds with acupuncture application.

Section Two describes the Short and Long-Term Application of magnetic therapy pads to problem areas of the body to increase energy flow and circulation and to stimulate the lymphatic system, thus bringing more oxygen and nutrients to the cells and tissues and speeding the elimination of toxic wastes and the healing of injuries. Both methods can be understood easily and used effectively by anyone, either professional or lay person, with the same results as those obtained by an experienced practitioner.

Section Two describes also the use and benefits of other Magnetic Field Therapy products for Total Body Wellness.

Numerous studies have established the effect of Magnetic Field Therapy on the human body. See the references listed at the end of this handbook, as well as those quoted in Section 3. The body heals itself over time, as many "permanent" ailments begin to correct themselves.

How Magnetic Fields Affect the Body
(from "An Overview of Biomagnetic Therapeutics"
By Edward A. Hacmac, D.C.)

[One] scientist whose comprehensive studies of magnetic fields and healing have been widely published is Physicist/ Psychologist Dr. Buryl Payne, inventor of the first biofeedback instruments and former professor at Boston University and Goddard College. His recent books, *The Body Magnetic* and *Getting Started in Magnetic Healing* have served as authoritative handbooks for professionals and lay people alike.

According to Dr. Payne, sensitive research instruments have allowed scientists to document some of the ways magnetic fields affect living organisms. He cites specific factors now known to be involved in magnetic healing. Among them are:

• Increased blood flow with resultant increased oxygen-carrying capacity, both of which are basic to helping the body heal itself;

• Changes in migration of calcium ions which can either bring calcium ions to heal a broken bone in half the usual time, or can help move calcium away from painful, arthritic joints;

• The pH balance (acid/alkaline) of various body fluids (often out of balance in conjunction with illness or abnormal conditions) can apparently be altered by magnetic fields;

• Hormone production from the endocrine glands can be either increased or decreased by magnetic stimulation;

• Altering of enzyme activity and other bio-chemical processes.

As an example of specific effects created when a magnetic field is applied to the body, below are typical changes that have been documented:

• Electricity is generated in blood vessels;
• Ionized particles increase in the blood;
• Autonomic nerves are excited;
• Circulation is improved.

To better understand the implications of providing the body with an adequate magnetic environment, it is important to understand the basic movement of certain body fluids and their role in health and disease.

In a somewhat simplified explanation, as the heart pumps approx-imately 80 times per minute, blood in the arteries forces nutrient-laden liquid through pores in the capillaries into the cell area to nourish the cells. (This liquid is called plasma while it is in the bloodstream and is re-named "lymph" once it leaves the bloodstream.)

The blood proteins in the vessels have a high affinity for water, and aid in pulling liquid back into the blood vessels. Through the venous system, the "used" blood is returned to the heart and lungs for purification and re-charging.

Because each individual cell, and the body as a whole, is an electrical generator, the cells must have oxygen to convert glucose into energy, and the balance of potassium/sodium within each cell must remain correct to keep the generators going.

The blood plasma contains numerous cells and protein molecules suspended in it. Under ordinary conditions, the normal blood pressure causes some of the blood proteins to continually seep through the tiny capillary pores into the spaces around the cells. There is not enough pressure in the cells to push these proteins back through the pores, so they must be continually removed and returned to the blood stream via the lymphatic system.

Pain and disease begin when conditions cause the capillary pores to dilate and allow the escape of significant quantities of blood proteins into the cellular area. This crowding of the proteins attracts fluid (inflammation), causes pain, and deprives some of the cells in the area of proper oxygen and nutrients, resulting in poor cellular functioning. These malfunctioning cells, if not carried away and disposed of by the lymphatic system, begin to destroy healthy cells and may keep proliferating into cancer or re-enter the bloodstream and cause leukemia.

If the lymphatic system completely fails to function and these blood proteins become trapped throughout the body, death can occur within hours.

According to Dr. C. Samuel West, chemist and internationally recognized lymphologist, trapped blood proteins are the one common denominator present in all pain and disease....

In citing circumstances which can cause trapped blood proteins, Dr. West lists the following: shallow breathing, improper exercise, shock, stress, anger, fear, tea, coffee, liquor, tobacco, drugs, salt, sugar, fat, high-cholesterol food, too much meat and others.

Many years of research and clinical application have shown that the simple introduction of a magnetic field can provide stimulation and enhancement of the lymphatic system, as well as every cell within the body. The magnetic field does not heal; it merely aids the cells in creating an optimum environment in which the body can begin to heal itself. Between the circulatory, lymphatic and neurological effects, outstanding advances in health can be obtained.

Many biomagnetic practitioners are now offering education, treatment, and magnetic devices to those seeking alternative health care. Among the most viable of these options is a magnetic sleep system developed in Japan. Users are able to sleep nightly within a cocoon of balanced magnetic energy to revitalize their bodies, with the system providing ongoing effectiveness levels.

Biomagnetic Research Continues

Around the world, research on the therapeutic potential of magnetism is continuing, and the publication, *Journal of Bioelectricity*, is devoted to the field. Among the places where this leading-edge technology is being studied are Loma Linda University in San Diego; New York University; the Massachusetts Institute of Technology; the Institute for Magnetotherapy in Madras, India; the University of Leeds in England; the University of Colorado; the University of South Carolina; the University of California at San Francisco; Columbia University in New York; Florida State University; and scores of other laboratories and institutions in Japan, Germany, Sweden and other nations.

The Healing Crisis

A healing crisis is in effect when the body is in the process of elimination. Reactions may be mild or they may be severe. One should expect this and work toward it. The body's inherent desire is perfect health. We have the ability to earn our way back to that state. The body must go through an elimination process to achieve good health. There will be ups and downs. One does not go immediately into good health. This elimination process we call the "healing process."

A healing crisis results when all body systems work in concert to eliminate waste products and set the stage for regeneration. Old tissues are replaced with new. A disease crisis, on the other hand, is not a natural one and works against the body's natural processes. Symptoms during a healing crisis may be identical to the disease, but there is an important difference—elimination. A cleansing, purifying process is underway and stored wastes are in a free-flowing state. Sometimes pain during the healing crisis is of greater intensity than when the chronic disease is building up. This may explain why there may be a brief flare-up in one's condition.

The crisis will usually bring about past conditions in whatever order the body is capable of handling them at the time. People often forget the disease or injuries they have had in the past, but are usually reminded during crisis. Reactions could include skin eruptions, nausea, headache, sleepiness, unusual fatigue, diarrhea, head or chest cold, ear infections, boils, or any other way the body uses to loosen and eliminate toxins. The crisis usually lasts three days, but if the energy of the patient is low it may last for a week or more. The body needs juices, and especially water, to help carry off the toxins. This is a time for rest—mental as well as physical rest.

One crisis is not always enough for a complete cure. The person in a chronic state, who has gone through many disease processes in life, must go through these processes again. Often the crisis will come after one feels his very best, setting the stage for the action. Most people feel an energy boost the first few days. Then toxins are dumped into the blood stream for elimination. Go as slowly as your body needs to so that your elimination is gradual and comfortable.

With a more serious condition there may be many small crises to go through before the final one is possible. Everything must be considered and given its proper place in the build-up to a healing crisis. One should expect it and work towards it.

Section 1

Magnetic Field Therapy

Acupressure Method

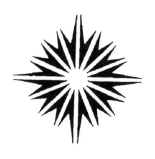

Procedures

In the Acupressure Method of Magnetic Field Therapy two magnetic therapy pads are held briefly on specific points along the acupressure meridians (energy channels) to increase and balance the flow of energy through the body. The magnetic therapy pad to be used is the Mini, which is about the size of a silver dollar and has a strength of 700 gauss, or the Maxi, which is 3 1/2" in diameter and has a strength of 650 gauss.

The procedures described in this section can be performed person-to-person or can be self-administered. Each of the recommended procedures is specifically related to certain ailments. The first stage, identified as "Greeting," is essential to the overall process. Do the Greeting first, followed by the procedure for "Metabolism," then go on to the specific procedure to treat the area or condition requiring attention.

Once a procedure has been completed and the healing process started, it is advisable to let the body have time to "cycle" before another treatment is administered. A minimum of one or two hours is adequate.

Cautions and Proper Usage

You may wish to discuss this therapy with your doctor. Certainly, a physician should be consulted concerning any serious problem. No medical claims are made for Magnetic Field Therapy nor are there any inferences that it is a substitute for conventional medical techniques. Magnetic Field Therapy is used to increase energy flow, relax tense muscles, relieve musculo-skeletal discomfort, and accelerate the body's own healing process by increasing blood flow and lymphatic circulation in the area under the influence of the magnet.

Magnets work differently on each individual. There is no guarantee expressed or implied that magnets will relieve your particular tension, relieve your particular pain, or accelerate the healing process for your particular injury. They work with varying results in varying time frames for each individual. You will need to experiment with the use, placement, and effect of the magnets on your problem area. The magnets may not be effective for you in all of the cited situations.

Under no condition should Magnetic Field Therapy be used by persons wearing cardiac pace-makers or defibrillators, since they are electromagnetically programmed. Wait 24 to 48 hours after suffering a sprain, hematoma, or wound before applying magnetic therapy pads. Adherence to the acronym RICE (R=Rest, I=Ice, C=Compression, E=Elevation) is best during this period to reduce swelling. It is recommended also that Magnetic Field Therapy not be used by women in the first trimester of pregnancy.

Do not allow credit cards, cassette tapes, video tapes, watches or other electronic equipment to come in contact with any magnetic product.

Do not stack one magnet on top of another, since the higher strength may increase the discomfort.

The magnetic therapy pads can be applied over light clothing or directly on the skin. Place the cloth side toward the body. Be sure the skin where you will be placing the magnets is clean. The cloth pads on the magnets will absorb ointments, rubs, Vaseline, or any other surface medication. (Note: Removal of the cloth pad will not harm the magnet. However, should yours wear out or become detached, adhesive-backed moleskin works very well as a replacement.)

Problem Areas or Conditions and Applicable Procedures

The following list shows the various problem areas or conditions which can be treated, together with the applicable procedures to use:

Problem Area or Condition	Use Procedures For:	Page
Allergy	infection	25
Alzheimer's disease	metabolism; head; neck	18, 23, 27
Angina pectoris	upper back; heart; lungs	20, 24, 26
Anxiety	psoriasis	28
Arm problems	neck; shoulder; local	27, 29
Arthritis	metabolism; local	18
Asthma	lungs; psoriasis	27,28
Blood pressure	upper back; heart	20,24
Broken bones	metabolism; local	18
Bronchitis	metabolism; infection; lungs	18, 25, 26
Bunions	metabolism; lower back; local	18, 20
Cancer	metabolism; upper back; local	18, 20
Cholesterol	metabolism	18
Circulation	heart	24
Colds and flu	upper back; infection; sinus	20, 25, 30
Colitis and constipation	abdomen; lower back	19, 20
Cystic fibrosis	metabolism; local	18
Cysts	metabolism; upper back; local	18, 20
Diabetes	metabolism; upper back	18, 20
Diverticulitis	abdomen; lower back	19, 20
Down's Syndrome	head; neck; local problems	23, 27

Note: **"Local" means where the pain is.**
To "work" means to hold the magnetic field therapy pad on the designated acupressure point.

Problem Area or Condition	Use Procedures For:	Page
Emphysema	upper back along spine; lungs	20, 25
Epilepsy	head	23
Fertility problems	abdomen; lower back (on men, work tailbone)	19, 20
Fingers (numb or tingle)	neck; shoulder; local	27, 29
Foot problems	lower back; local	20
Glaucoma	metabolism; eyes	18, 22
Gout	metabolism; local	18
Headaches	head; neck	23, 27
Heart problems	heart	24
Hemorrhoids	abdomen; lower back (tailbone)	19, 20
Hernia	abdomen; lower back	19, 20
Hiatal hernia	solar plexus	31
Hormone troubles	abdomen; lower back	19, 20
Hypoglycemia	metabolism	18
Indigestion	solar plexus	31
Infection	infection	25
Influenza	infection	25
Knee and leg problems	lower back; local	20
Leukemia	metabolism; upper back; solar plexus	18, 20, 31
Lupus	metabolism; upper back; infection; local	18, 20, 25
Menopause	abdomen; lower back	19, 20
Menstrual problems	abdomen	19
Migraine headaches	head; neck	23, 27
Multiple sclerosis	metabolism; whole back; head; neck	18,20,23,27
Nervous stomach	psoriasis; solar plexus	28, 31

Problem Area or Condition	Use Procedures For:	Page
Paget's disease	back	20
Parkinson's disease	head; neck (repeatedly)	23, 27
Pelvic injury	back	20
Pneumonia	metabolism; upper back; infection; lungs	18, 20, 25, 26
Pregnancy (to ease delivery)	abdomen; lower back	19, 20
Psoriasis	psoriasis	28
Sciatica	lower back	20
Scoliosis	metabolism; entire back	18, 20
Shingles	psoriasis	28
Shoulder	shoulder	29
Sinus	sinus	30
Solar plexus	solar plexus	31
Stress	psoriasis	28
Stroke	upper back; head; heart; neck	20, 23, 24, 27
Tumors	metabolism; upper back; local	18, 20
Ulcers	psoriasis; solar plexus	28, 31
Urinary tract and prostate	abdomen; lower back	19, 20
Varicose veins	metabolism; lower back; heart; local	18, 20, 24
Warts	metabolism; local	18

To begin, do the "Greeting," then the "Metabolism," and then proceed to the area requiring attention. Problems of a serious nature can be addressed every hour or two. For maintenance and continued relief, apply as needed.

The purpose of the greeting is
to establish the magnetic
harmony of the body.

Use Dominant Hand
Step 1 - Hold point **1** for 6 seconds with magnet
Step 2 - Hold point **2** for 6 seconds with magnet

Step 1 - Use magnets to work points **1**
through **3**, for 6 seconds each.
Repeat 3 times.

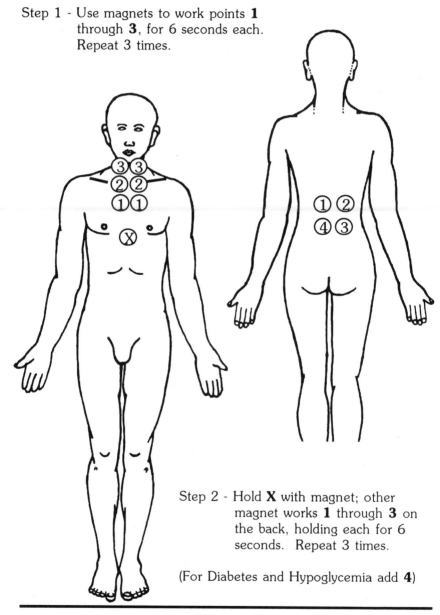

Step 2 - Hold **X** with magnet; other
magnet works **1** through **3** on
the back, holding each for 6
seconds. Repeat 3 times.

(For Diabetes and Hypoglycemia add **4**)

Step 1 - Hold **X** with magnet; other magnet works **1** through **5**, for 6 seconds each.

Step 2 - Hold **T** point on "Back" chart at sacrum "triangle;" with other magnet work **1** through **5** and **X** for 6 seconds each.

Step 3 - With two magnets work **1** & **X**; **2** & **3**; **4** & **5**, for 6 seconds each.

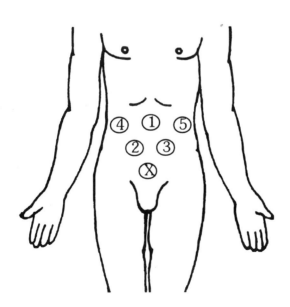

Back

Step 1 - Hold **X** with magnet on coccyx (tailbone); hold 2 magnets at base of skull at point **1** for 6 seconds.*

Step 2 - Continuing to hold at point **X**, hold other magnet at point **2** at center of base of skull for 6 seconds.

Step 3 - Hold **T** with a magnet; other magnet works points **3** through **9** for 6 seconds each.

Step 4 - With 2 magnets work points **10** - **17** for 6 seconds each (approximately every other vertebra).

Step 5 - When magnets are at point **17** on both sides of the spine, draw them smoothly and slowly in a single sweep down to points **10**, curving them gently outward and lifting off.

*Only place in handbook where 3 magnets are required. Step can be completed by holding on point **1** on right side for 6 seconds, and moving to point **1** on left side for 6 seconds.

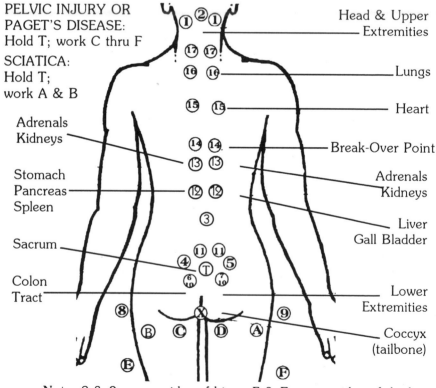

PELVIC INJURY OR PAGET'S DISEASE:
Hold T; work C thru F

SCIATICA:
Hold T;
work A & B

Adrenals
Kidneys

Stomach
Pancreas
Spleen

Sacrum

Colon
Tract

Head & Upper Extremities

Lungs

Heart

Break-Over Point

Adrenals
Kidneys

Liver
Gall Bladder

Lower Extremities

Coccyx (tailbone)

Note: 8 & 9 are on sides of hips. E & F are on sides of thighs.

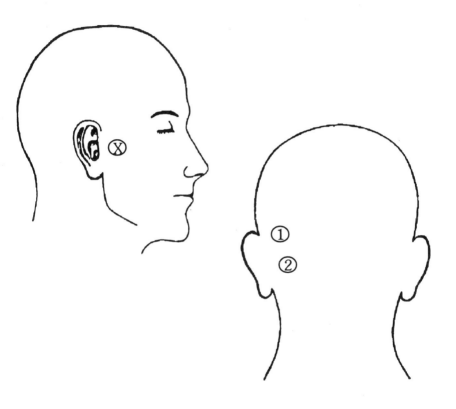

Step 1 - Hold **X** with magnet; other magnet works **1** and **2** on same side for 6 seconds then reverse sides for 6 seconds.

Step 2 - Work **X** on both sides of head; then **1** on both sides; then **2** on both sides, for 6 seconds each.

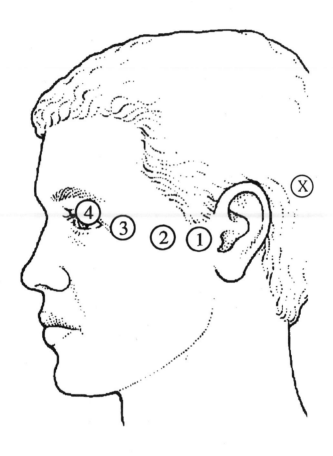

Step 1 - Hold **X** with magnet (behind ear at first dent above rise); other magnet works **1** through **4** on the same side for 6 seconds.

Step 2 - Reverse sides and repeat this set.

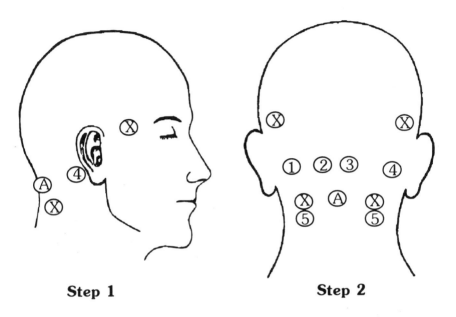

Step 1   **Step 2**

Step 1 - With finger on **X** beside the eye, hold magnet on lower **X** with thumb; work **A** for 6 seconds. Repeat procedure on other side of head.

Step 2 - Place one finger from each hand on two top **X**'s. Hold magnet on one lower **X** with thumb while other magnet works opposite side **1** through **5** for 6 seconds each. Keep fingers on top **X**'s. Then, holding magnet on other lower **X** with thumb, work other side **1** through **5** for 6 seconds each.

Step 3 - With two magnets work the left and right sides at the same time, points **1** - **5**, for 6 seconds each.

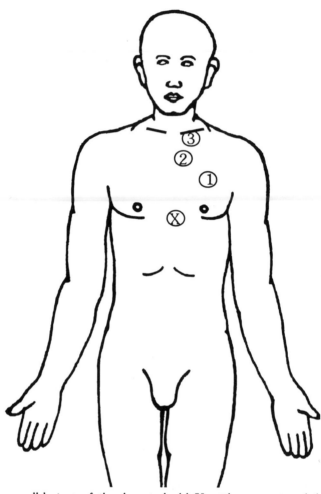

For major well-being of the heart, hold **X** with magnet, while other magnet works points **1** and **2** for 6 seconds each.   Repeat 3 times. For circulation, veins, and blood pressure, hold **X** with magnet, while other magnet works **3**.   Hold for 6 seconds.   Repeat 3 times.

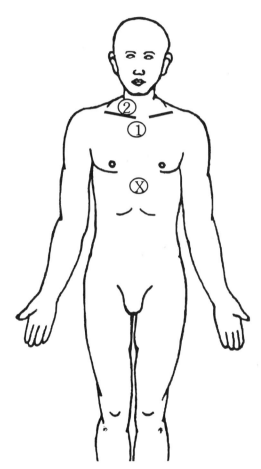

Infection, Influenza:
Hold **X** with magnet; with other magnet work **1** for 6 seconds.

Allergy:
Hold **X** with magnet; with other magnet work **2** for 6 seconds. Repeat 3 times.

Lungs

Oxygen Control Gland.

Step 1 - Hold **X** with magnet; other
magnet works **1** through **6**,
for 6 seconds each.

Step 2 - Use magnets at **1** and **4**;
2 and **5**; **3** and **6**, for 6
seconds each.

Repeat each step 3 times, holding each
point for 6 seconds.

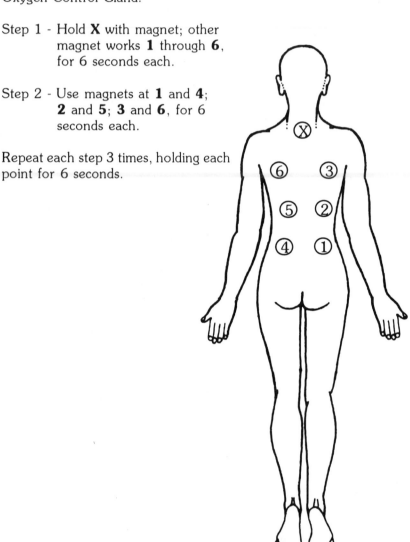

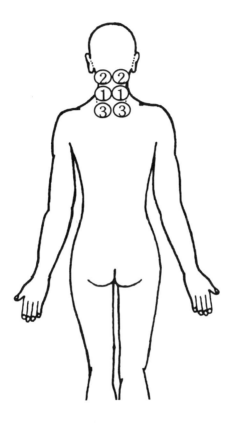

With two magnets work **1** through **3** for 6 seconds each.
Repeat 3 times.

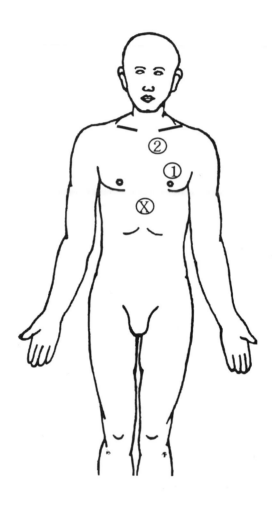

Hold **X** with magnet; other magnet works **1** and **2** for 6 seconds each.
Repeat 3 times.

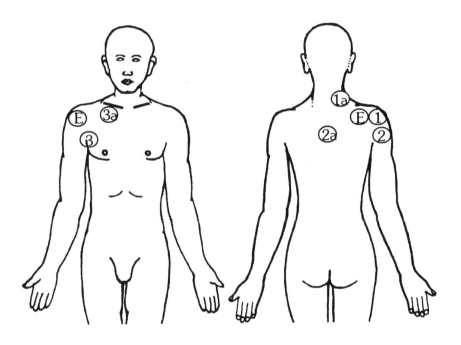

Step 1 - Hold magnet at **1**; use other magnet to sweep from 1 up line **1a** and down to **E**.

Step 2 - Hold magnet at **2**; use other magnet to sweep from 2 across line **2a** and up to **E**.

Step 3 - Hold magnet at **3**; use other magnet to sweep from 3 up line **3a** and across to **E**.

1 is the tip of the shoulder.
2 is indentation below back shoulder.
3 is indentation below front shoulder.

Sinus

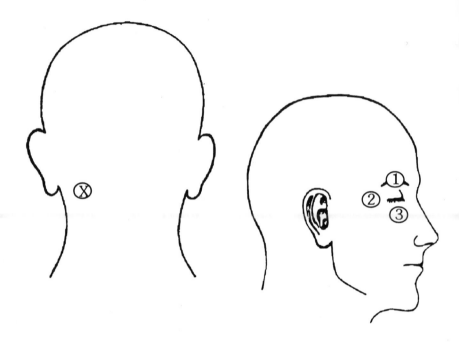

Step 1 - Hold **X** with magnet on left side; other magnet works **1**, **2**, and **3** on right side for 6 seconds each.

Step 2 - Hold **X** with magnet on right side; other magnet works **1**, **2** and **3** on left side. Hold each work point for 6 seconds.

Step 3 - Hold both **X** points with magnets for 6 seconds. Hold both **1** points with magnets for 6 seconds. Hold both **2** points with magnets for 6 seconds. Hold both **3** points with magnets for 6 seconds.

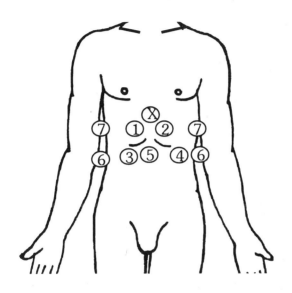

Step 1 - Hold **X** with magnet; other magnet works **1** through **7** for 6 seconds each.

Step 2 - Hold magnet just below ribs, while other magnet works **1** through **7** and **X** for 6 seconds each.

Step 3 - With two magnets work **1** & **2**; **3** & **4**; **X** & **5**, **6**'s & **7**'s for 6 seconds each.

Note: **6** & **7** are on sides of torso.

Section 2

Magnetic Field Therapy

Short and Long-Term

Application

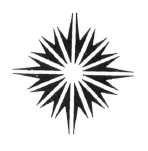

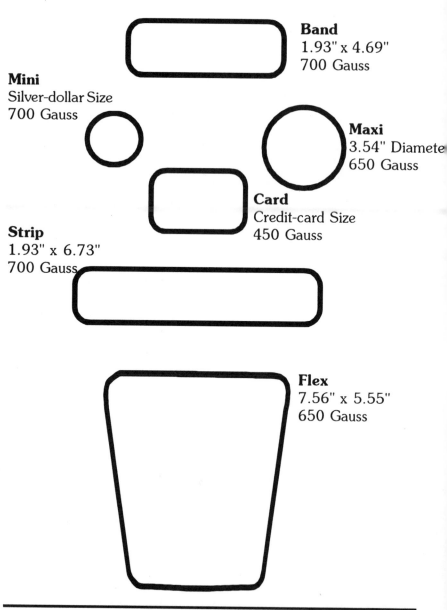

Band
1.93" x 4.69"
700 Gauss

Mini
Silver-dollar Size
700 Gauss

Maxi
3.54" Diamete
650 Gauss

Card
Credit-card Size
450 Gauss

Strip
1.93" x 6.73"
700 Gauss

Flex
7.56" x 5.55"
650 Gauss

Use of Flexible Magnetic Therapy Pads

Flexible magnetic therapy pads can also be used very effectively without reference to the points along the acupressure meridians. However, in this case the pads must be left in place for a longer period of time. The pads are placed over the area of discomfort or at the point of origin of the pain.

The Band, Card, Flex, Maxi, Mini, and Strip are designed to be used any time and any place to relieve muscular aches and pains and to relieve tension in the body. These patented pads, of positive and negative alternating polarity, cause the blood vessels to widen and thus increase the blood flow to the affected area. They also stimulate the lymphatic system. The body's own healing processes are accelerated by the increased concentration of oxygen and vital nutrients and the simultaneous removal of toxic waste products that result from injured tissue.

The use of the magnetic therapy pads is simple; just follow the suggestions to ensure proper results. The flexibility of the pads allows them to fit into everyone's life-style with the greatest of comfort. They can be cut to shape without losing their magnetic properties.

Cautions and Proper Usage

You may wish to discuss this therapy with your doctor. Certainly, a physician should be consulted concerning any serious problem. No medical claims are made for Magnetic Field Therapy nor are there any inferences that it is a substitute for conventional medical techniques. Magnetic Field Therapy is used to increase energy flow, relax tense muscles, relieve musculo-skeletal discomfort, and accelerate the body's own healing process by increasing blood flow and lymphatic circulation in the area under the influence of the magnet.

Magnets work differently on each individual. There is no guarantee expressed or implied that magnets will relieve your particular tension, relieve your particular pain, or accelerate the healing process for your particular injury. They work with varying results in varying time frames for each individual. You will need to experiment with the use, placement, and effect of the magnets on your problem area. The magnets may not be effective for you in all of the cited situations.

Under no condition should Magnetic Field Therapy be used by persons wearing cardiac pace-makers or defibrillators, since they are electromagnetically programmed. Wait 24 to 48 hours after suffering a sprain, hematoma, or wound before applying magnetic therapy pads. Adherence to the acronym RICE (R=Rest, I=Ice, C=Compression, E=Elevation) is best during this period to reduce swelling. It is recommended also that Magnetic Field Therapy not be used by women in the first trimester of pregnancy.

Do not stack one magnet on top of another, since the higher strength may increase the discomfort.

Do not place credit cards, cassette tapes, video tapes, watches or other electronic equipment on any magnetic products.

The magnetic therapy pads can be applied over light clothing or directly on the skin. Place the cloth side toward the body. Be sure the skin where you will be placing the magnets is clean. The cloth pads on the magnets will absorb ointments, rubs, Vaseline, or any other surface medication. (Note: Removal of the cloth pad will not harm the magnet. However, should yours wear out or become detached, adhesive-backed moleskin works very well as a replacement.)

To hold the magnetic therapy pads in place, use a knitted wristband or headband, elastic bandage (never neoprene), or paper tape for sensitive skin. Surgical tape is best (e.g., 3M Micropore tape, Curity's Tenderskin, or Dermicel by Johnson & Johnson). Avoid adhesive or Scotch tape, as these may remove the gold plating from the surface of the magnetic therapy pads.

A strip of male Velcro (spiked side) stuck to the back of a pad will hold the pad firmly in place inside a bandage or knitted band.

If you wish to remove the Velcro later, wrap the pad in plastic before applying the Velcro.

If possible, wear the pads 24 hours a day, removing them only when bathing. Water will not hurt the pads; in fact, they can be washed, but it is inadvisable to leave a wet pad next to the skin.

Suggestions for Short and Long-Term Application of Magnetic Field Therapy

Ankle

Card or Maxi

For fresh sprains, ice is used for the first 24 to 48 hours. Use a pad with male Velcro inside an Ace or similar ankle support. Continue to use for two days after discomfort is gone.

Arthritis

Card, Maxi, Mini, Band, Strip or Flex

See instructions for the affected joint(s). Overall relief from arthritis pain may be enhanced by use of the magnetic *mattress pads, pillows, seat cushions, massage balls,* and *insoles* described at the end of this section.

Maxi

Wear a Maxi on the chest. Women can tuck one into their bra. A strip or two of male Velcro on the back of the pad will make it cling to a man's undershirt. Or place the pad inside a replacement pocket and fasten the flap over a chain or cord worn around the neck.

Back (High & Low)

Card, Maxi, Mini, Band, Strip or Flex

On the high back, the discomfort is nearly always a few inches from the spine to the right, to the left or both. In all cases, you will be able to find that area which is the most tender. Any of the pads mentioned can be used depending upon the size of the affected area. Always use one pad on each side of the high back, even if the discomfort is only on one side. If you treat only one side, the other side will compensate and a problem will be created where none previously existed. Affix the pads with flexible tape. Or, stick male Velcro to the back of the pads and position them inside an undershirt or T-shirt.

For the lower back, the pads are taped over the areas of most discomfort, again on both sides. In addition, a pad can be taped to the center of the lower back right over the spine. Men should take their wallets or any other items out of the rear pockets as these put pressure on the sciatic nerve, which makes the condition worse. Women can find the areas in the lower back easily by looking for the slight depressions at the base of the back and above the buttocks. Place a magnetic therapy pad in each of those depressions with flexible tape.

A Flex may be used in place of any of the other pads. It covers a larger area and has Velcro strips attached to its rear surface so you can place it inside clothing and it won't shift around. It is especially useful for low-back pain. Care should be taken when going to the bathroom that you don't forget it is there and let it fall into the water. Since the Velcro can tear knitted underwear and pantyhose, you may wish to wear the Flex between your underwear and your outer clothing rather than next to the skin.

Bags under the Eyes

Mini

This procedure may be used to temporarily reduce or eliminate bags under the eyes. This can be done every morning for as little as 20 minutes or up to an hour. Cut a Mini in half and warm the two halves between your hands for at least fifteen seconds. Lie down with your head on a pillow. Gently bend the pieces of the Mini so they touch all the skin directly below the eye. Relax your facial muscles and close your eyes. Gently place half a Mini with the flat side towards the eye, so that it is barely touching the lower eyelash. You may have to reshape the half Mini, as it is important that all areas touch the skin. Do not use tape or pressure to keep the pad in place. You may want to try this on only one eye first to be able to see the difference. Both eyes should then be done at the same time. It should be noted that this does not permanently remove bags under the eyes.

Carpal Tunnel Syndrome

Mini, Band or Strip

The nerve running through the inside of the forearm and through the carpal tunnel gets trapped by swollen tissue (caused by repetitive motion/stress, scar tissue or fibrous ligaments), sometimes causing pain in the hand, fingers or even the forearm and elbow. This problem is common in people who use constant and repetitious hand and finger motions throughout the day. Using flexible tape or Ace bandage, secure one Mini over the center of the wrist on the inside where the nerve is trapped and another on the outside of the wrist. Or, for maximum effect, wrap a Band or Strip completely around the wrist. It may take several days to experience a reduction in pain or it may take several weeks. The pads should continue to be worn for four to five weeks.

Feet

Top of Foot or Top of the Toes

Card, Maxi, Mini, Band or Strip

Use flexible tape to tape the pad of choice to these areas and continue for two days after discomfort is gone.

Bottom of Foot

Card

With flexible tape, fasten the Card to the bottom of the foot at night or whenever you go to sleep, or wear the Card inside a pair of socks. Your feet will feel great in the morning.

Because the bottom of the foot is richly endowed with blood vessels and nerve endings, the stronger magnetic field of the other magnets may cause discomfort. However, if the Card is not effective, you may wish to try the stronger pads. Magnetic *insoles*, another magnetic therapy product, may be worn during the day or evening to increase circulation in the feet and legs. They may also alleviate or eliminate night-time leg cramps.

Hand Joints

Card or Maxi

The hand requires the use of two pads, one on top of and one directly below the fingers. They are either taped on with flexible tape or placed inside a tight mitten so that the pads are very close to the skin. The best time for this use is at home at a time when it is possible to leave them on for long periods without removing them to wash the hands. Use of this procedure is recommended while sleeping for best results. In the hand, the discomfort may never disappear completely, so a continual program of at least one to two hours at night may have to be followed.

Magnetic *massage balls* may also be used to relieve discomfort in the hand joints. Take the *balls* out of their case and roll them in your hand. Or wear them inside a pair of gloves while you sleep. The magnetic field in the *balls* will increase circulation in the hands and help to relieve pain, including arthritis pain. Additionally, the *massage balls* can be used to stimulate the reflexology points in your hand, which helps to relieve tension and also to keep you alert. (To open the case, squeeze the ends, not the sides.)

Hips

Card, Maxi, or Flex

Tape either a Card or Maxi to the joint area in the hip first and then to any other area that you feel radiating discomfort. Always position the flexible tape in the ways that the stretch has the most benefit. Or wear the pad in your hip pocket. (Be sure to remove your wallet.) Continue use for one week after discomfort is gone.

A Flex may be used in place of the other pads. It covers a larger area and has Velcro strips on the back so you can place it inside clothing and it will stay in place. Care should be taken when going to the bathroom that you don't forget it is there and let it fall into the water. Since the Velcro can tear knitted underwear and pantyhose, you may wish to wear the Flex between your underwear and your outer clothing rather than next to the skin.

Knees

Mini, Band or Strip

To place the magnet properly on the knee, sit down, expose the knee and straighten your leg forward. As you do so you will see a depression on either side of your knee cap. You should use two pads, one in each depression in conjunction with a knee brace. An elastic knee brace is made by Ace and has side stabilizers. The knee brace is pulled up over the leg so half is above the knee and half below. The magnets are then placed under the brace in the two depressions. Male Velcro applied to the back of the pads will help keep them in place. The pads and brace should be worn for at least a week, or even longer, after the discomfort is gone.

Menstrual Cramps

Mini, Band or Strip

Place a magnet over each ovary just below the bikini line. Use flexible tape to hold them in place.

Neck

Card or Maxi

During the day, place the pad of choice over the center of the area on the neck and affix with flexible tape. At night for maximum benefit, a pad can be fastened to a cervical collar by attaching a piece of male Velcro to the gold surface. The collar is then placed around the neck in the usual manner. Remember that the pad must be close to the skin. It may be better for the pad to be first taped to the neck followed by the cervical collar. By not moving the neck at night, we allow the body, with the aid of the magnets, to do its job. Two days of use are recommended after the discomfort is gone.

The magnetic field strength of the Mini, Band and Strip may be too strong for use on the neck, but if the Card or Maxi is not effective, you may wish to try these stronger pads. Sleeping on a magnetic *pillow* may also relieve the pain of arthritis or muscle strain in the neck.

Phantom Limb Pain

Card, Maxi, Mini, Band or Strip

Phantom limb pain is caused by severed nerve endings continuing to send pain signals to the brain. Place a magnet right on the end of the stump and keep it there for at least thirty minutes after the cessation of pain.

Shoulder Pain

Card, Maxi, Mini, Band, or Strip

Often the pain in a shoulder radiates down from the side of the arm between the biceps and the triceps but the source of the pain is actually on your shoulder. In fact, the source is closer to your neck rather than the arm where the discomfort is prominent. To locate this area so you can best find the appropriate spot, take off your shirt and stand facing a mirror. Extend your hand straight up in the air over your head and you will see a valley between the round part of your shoulder and your neck. It is in this valley you should place the magnetic pad of choice. The pad should be secured with flexible tape (the Card, Strip and Band should be secured with the long part going from front to back). If, after two days, there is still discomfort in the higher part of the arm or lower shoulder, place another pad on that area with flexible tape but always keep the first pad on the primary area. Use of the pads in these areas should continue for one week after the discomfort is gone. These areas are heavy muscle areas and require more care.

Sleeping on a magnetic *pillow* may also help relieve shoulder pain.

Sinus Headaches

Card or Maxi

A Card or Maxi may be used to relieve a sinus headache by holding it up to your forehead or over the eyebrows or under the eyes for approximately 20 minutes or until the pain is gone. A headband may be used to hold the magnets in place.

The magnetic field strength of the Mini, Band and Strip in some instances may be too strong and cause discomfort, but if the Card or Maxi is not effective, you may wish to try these stronger pads.

Mini, Band or Strip

Stress headaches are caused by tension in the shoulder muscles that go up the neck and are attached to the base of the skull. A flexible magnetic therapy pad may relieve the tension in the muscle, thereby relieving the headache. To find the best spot to relieve tension in the shoulder muscle, use your right hand to feel along the left shoulder muscle to find the motor point (aka: release point or trigger point), a hard pebble of muscle between the spine and the shoulder blade. Place a magnet over that motor point and over the motor point on the right side. Use flexible tape to hold the pad in place.

A magnet can also be used right on the neck muscle at the base of the skull. The extra strength of the Mini, Band and Strip may cause dizziness or other discomfort if used on the neck. For this reason you may wish to use a Card or Maxi, or place one of the other pads lower on the neck.

Temporal Mandibular Joint

Card, Maxi, Mini, Band, or Strip

The nerve in the temporal mandibular joint (TMJ) can be the source of considerable pain for some people. Place one of the magnetic therapy pads over the joint to relieve pain. A headband may be used to hold the magnet in place. Since this pain is nerve related, it may be necessary to keep the magnet in place for an extended period of time to achieve results.

The magnetic field strength of a Mini, Band or Strip may be too strong and cause discomfort, but if the Card or Maxi is not effective, you may wish to try these stronger pads.

Tennis, Racquet Ball or Squash Elbow

Mini, Band or Strip

Although we say to locate the central point of maximum pain, that is not so easy in this situation. The pain from this form of tendonitis radiates down the forearm, but the actual source of the problem is the elbow. To determine the appropriate placement of a pad hold your arm straight in front of you and turn your hand so that the palm of your hand is facing out and your thumb is pointing down. You will now see a small depression above your elbow joint. That is the exact point—no higher or lower, even if the pain is in another area above or more often below. Using an Ace elbow bandage, pull the bandage over the arm until half is above the elbow and half is below. The right size bandage is important for comfort as well as circulation. Now take the pad of choice and slide it into the bandage over the small depression. To keep the pad from shifting in the bandage, you may want to attach a piece of male Velcro on top of the gold surface of the magnet. You can wear this all day and night, only taking it off to shower or bathe. How long it is used is different in every individual; however, it should be worn at least two days after all discomfort has disappeared.

Thumb

Card or Maxi

Using flexible tape, place one of the pads half on the top of the hand and half on the bottom, covering the fleshy area at the base of the thumb which is part of the palm of the hand. You must tape it so that you have immobilized the thumb. The only way the thumb will get better is if it cannot be moved. This is in most cases a long process depending upon the age of the injury. Use the pad day and night, taking it off only to shower or bathe. Continue use for a week after discomfort is gone. Because we use the thumb for so many things, to insure that you do not reinjure the area, we add one week rather than two days.

Wrinkles on the Face

Card or Maxi

For large areas of wrinkles, use a Card or Maxi on each side of the face. Use this procedure at home so that the pads can be left in place overnight or for at least a few hours. It should be noted that this does not permanently remove wrinkles.

Wrist Strains

Card, Maxi, Mini, Band, or Strip

Slide the magnetic pad of choice into a wrist sweat band or Ace wrist elastic bandage. You will need the added stability of the wrist wrap to allow the pad to produce its maximum effect. To keep the pad from shifting use the same Velcro technique suggested for tennis elbow. Continue use at least two days after all discomfort has disappeared.

Magnetic Field Therapy for Total Body Wellness

In addition to using Magnetic Field Therapy to relieve local stress and discomfort, you can experience its benefits for your total body wellness by sleeping on a magnetic *mattress* or *mattress pad* and *pillow* and sitting on a magnetic *seat cushion*. They stimulate the circulatory and lymphatic systems, as well as balancing the energy flow, thus improving overall body functioning. According to Dr. Edward A. Hacmac, D.C., "when the body is placed within such a magnetic sleep system, kinesiology (muscle strength) testing shows each acupuncture meridian in the body is functioning in harmony within fifteen minutes. It logically follows that the longer a body remains in this environment, the more quickly it can balance itself."

Magnetic *mattresses*, *mattress pads*, and *pillows* are designed to provide a sound and restful sleep, so that one awakens with more energy and greater alertness. They reinforce the effect of the flexible magnetic therapy *pads*. For the bedridden they help to prevent bed sores. The magnets in these products have a strength of 800 gauss. A clinical test of magnetic *mattress pads* showed positive results in an average of 80% of cases of neck and shoulder pain, back pain, lower limb pain, insomnia, and fatigue (see Section 3).

A magnetic *seat cushion* with attached back is especially valuable for persons who are unable to exercise or who sit for long periods during the day. Persons who work with computers often desire the benefit of the magnetic field provided by the *seat cushion*. The *seat* can be taken along on trips and used for sleeping as well as sitting, so that you have the benefit of Magnetic Field Therapy even when away from home. Remove wallet from hip pocket to prevent the demagnetizing of credit cards. The strength of the magnets in the *seat cushion* is 800 gauss.

Keeping yourself in a beneficial magnetic field during the day and all night long brings harmony and balance to your body, so that you feel better and function better, both physically and mentally.

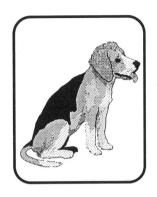

Pets enjoy the positive effects of Magnetic Field Therapy obtained from resting on the *seat cushions, mattresses, and mattresses pads*, and magnetic therapy products are beneficial in the care of horses (*see* Section 3).

Two other magnetic products contribute to total body wellness:

Magnetic *massage balls*, two 800-gauss magnetic *balls* in a case, can be used to give a relaxing massage to the entire body or to direct magnetic force to specific areas. The massage should be light but rapid. The faster the *balls* spin, the stronger the magnetic pulse and the deeper the penetration. When the *balls* are removed from the case and rolled in the hand, the specially designed nodules on the surface stimulate the reflexology points on the hand, thus stimulating the corresponding organs of the body, relieving stress, and promoting mental alertness. You can also put the *balls* on the floor and roll your feet over them. To open the case, squeeze the ends, not the sides. When you replace the *balls* in the case, be sure the circle inscribed on each *ball* faces up. When the second *ball* is inserted, the first *ball* will revolve, so the circle on it faces down.

Magnetic *insoles*, with a strength of 350 gauss, increase energy flow and stimulate the circulation in the feet and legs, thus benefitting the whole body. They can be worn during all or part of the day and/or during the evening. There are two kinds of magnetic *insoles*, those with a smooth surface and those covered with massage nodules which stimulate the reflexology points on the feet, thus stimulating the corresponding organs of the body, with a positive effect on overall well-being. Try both sides of the *insoles with the nodules* to see which works better for you. The *insoles* may also alleviate or eliminate night-time leg cramps.

According to Dr. H. L. Bansal, the drinking of magnetized water contributes to total body wellness by helping to regulate the acid-alkaline balance and the amount of bile in the digestive tract. It also improves intestinal motility so that toxic wastes which have accumulated in the colon are loosened and eliminated, soothes the nerves, and improves circulation by stimulating the ions in the blood stream. Used externally, magnetized water is beneficial for small wounds, eczema, and irritated eyes.

To magnetize a pint or a quart of distilled or other uncontaminated water or any other liquid, place it in a glass or plastic container with a nonmetallic cover. Set the container on any of the magnetic therapy pads described in this handbook for one or two hours with the cloth side of the pad up. Smaller amounts of liquid require less time. Drink an eight-ounce glass twice a day—before breakfast and dinner—in addition to your regular intake of water. Magnetized olive oil can be used externally to treat rheumatism and gout.

For more information on using magnetized substances to cleanse the body and promote healing, consult the book, *Magnetic Cure for Common Diseases*, by Dr. H. L. Bansal and Dr. R. S. Bansal.

Section 3

Articles and Excerpts Concerning Magnetic Field Therapy

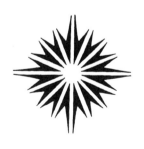

Magnetism is poised to revolutionize arthritis treatment. Donut-shaped machines soon may render aspirin and other anti-inflammatory drugs obsolete, at least as far as aching joints go.

Quiet research over the past quarter-century demonstrates that magnetic energy can produce helpful biological effects in human tissue, says Richard Markoll, a doctor and biophysicist who spent 24 years as a senior researcher at the University of Munich Teaching Hospital in Germany.

Patented rings. Now back in the U.S., the Long Island, New York, scientist is testing his patented invention—hi-tech rings that produce therapeutic magnetic fields.

People with arthritis, mainly osteoarthritis, place their aching joints inside the rings for 30 or 60 minutes, until they've spent a total of nine hours over three weeks inside the rings. Then, they resume their lives minus pain.

The method, which Markoll calls biomagnetic therapy, could replace much of conventional arthritis treatment, which relies on aspirin and other nonsteroidal anti-inflammatory drugs (NSAIDS) as a first line of treatment, and stronger measures such as steroids, gold injections and various types of surgery.

Extensive investigation of biomagnetic therapy shows that not only is it effective, says Markoll, but it's free of toxicity and side effects. "Patients call it a miracle cure," says Markoll. "I don't. Miracle is not a scientific term and I'm a scientist. But I do know that the pain relief is profound and that it lasts. And it causes no harm," he told *Your Health*.

Biomagnetic therapy. Markoll's specific field of expertise is pulsed electromagnetic fields (PEMF). His research convinced him that the abstractions he found so intriguing could help people. He developed practical applications through clinical investigation. The result is biomagnetic therapy.

His machines stimulate the growth, repair and healing of cartilage with low-energy PEMF. "We believe it causes new cartilage to grow. But we can't state that with absolute certainty yet because we don't perform exploratory surgery and look into the joint afterward. That would be the only way to verify that at present.

"But from lab experiments, we do know that PEMF stimulates the growth of bovine cartilage. By applying PEMF to a tissue culture of bovine cartilage, we have demonstrated an exponential repair or healing rate of the cartilage," he explains. "We'd like to think that's what's happening in humans, too. If we're right, that would explain the benefits. In effect, the treatment puts a new layer of cartilage into the joint."

A technique developed at the teaching hospital of the University of Wurzburg in Germany called dual energy absorptometry may allow Markoll to confirm his hypothesis. A computer software program runs two different X-ray systems, low-energy and high-energy, "and it allows you to differentiate the different anatomical structures in the joint. We plan to demonstrate what we think is happening—in about six months, we'll know definitely.

"In the meantime, we can state with certainty that we treat people and three weeks later they have no pain. And it lasts. We have treated people two, three, four and five years ago and they're still in great shape," Markoll noted. The technique is in an advanced investigational stage at this time. Thousands of patients have received the treatment so far. In the last two years alone, of the nearly 2,000 people who've have had it, 80 percent have shown significant improvement. Results of a controlled clinical trial have been published recently in the *Journal of Rheumatology*.

Trial results. In that trial, 27 patients with osteoarthritis received treatment; of those, 25 completed the month-long PEMF treatment. All patients experienced a 23- to 61-percent average improvement in pain, swelling and range of motion. Another group was treated with a placebo method for purposes of comparison. Their average improvement was only 2 to 18 percent.

The machines come in different sizes and types, depending upon which joints they're designed to treat—limbs, neck or back.

They consist of a magnetic field generator that creates low-powered magnetic fields via low-voltage, fluctuating direct current. This magnetic current runs through a "freely moving air coil" surrounding the joint being treated. The coil encircles the affected area but doesn't touch it during treatment.

Treatment lasts three or four weeks for a total of nine hours exposure to PEMF through the rings, either in 18 half-hour sessions or nine 60-minute sessions.

A recent, independent scientific discovery may help explain how or why Markoll's system works. Dr. Joseph Kirschvink, a geobiologist at California Institute of Technology, found tiny magnetite crystals inside human brain cells in autopsy experiments. The crystals are a compound of iron and oxygen and are highly magnetic. Other iron compounds in the body aren't magnetic. This is the first verification of the source of magnetic energy in humans.

Offers explanation. "Physicists and biophysicists have had trouble understanding how electromagnetic fields could affect human tissue until now. So what this discovery offers is another whole category of mechanisms that have not been considered," says Kirschvink.

The scientist's discovery has lent credibility to claims that power lines and other strong sources of electromagnetic fields might be harmful to human beings and suggests how harm might occur. But it could also help explain how and why Markoll's discovery helps people.

As far as Markoll is concerned, any solid information in the field of electromagnetic fields is helpful. But the science is already there to justify his therapy.

"Using magnets to treat people is one of the most controversial subjects in modern medicine," he says. "Although it has been dismissed as quackery, strong scientific studies exist which describe the mechanism by which it works. Many orthodox physicians and scientists worldwide have accepted this evidence."

Magnets are what make MRIs work, he points out (MRI stands

for magnetic resonance imaging, by the way). "Indeed, the use of magnetic fields to manipulate hydrogen atoms in the body is central to the imaging systems now in use," he adds.

Mimicking body's magnetism. "All living creatures produce magnetic fields, and there are theories that the interaction of different fields can affect the cell's ability to absorb calcium and other minerals. What we're doing is mimicking the body's own magnetic field, signalling the cell, or the DNA in cells, to do what it's supposed to do. Evidence also exists that pulsed magnetic fields can modulate the actions of hormones, antibodies and neurotransmitters."

The Food and Drug Administration is expected soon to approve the device (which Markoll invented and for which he holds the patent) for pre-market tests on 1,700 patient joints in the U.S. and 1,000 joints treated in Europe.

The final application for commercial approval is on file with the FDA pending those results, Markoll says. He expects to get the green light in about a year. Currently, the FDA considers his machines to be "nonsignificant risk" devices. This has meant trials of the devices have been able to proceed with a minimum of red tape and federal oversight until this point.

At present he is treating only osteoarthritis, but Markoll anticipates other applications. He expects the method will work for osteoporosis, rapid healing of recent injuries to the musculoskeletal system (including fractures, breaks, ligament, tendon and cartilage tears and muscle pulls) and even nerve damage caused by diabetes.

The Arthritis Foundation, the mouthpiece of conventional arthritis medicine, is aware of Markoll's work and neither endorses nor decries it until further studies are completed. It is interesting to ponder, however, what their position might be if one day Markoll's devices put a huge portion of conventional arthritis medicine out of business.

NOTE: This article describes the treatment of arthritis with magnetic therapy equipment located in a clinic or hospital. The flexible magnetic therapy pads and other products described in this *Magnetic Field Therapy Handbook* can be worn or used at home or in the course of one's normal activities outside of the home. An average of 80% of users of the products report positive results in relieving arthritis pain.

Summary of Beneficial Influence of Magnetic Therapy
From *Magnetic Therapy*
By Dr. H. L. Bansal

When a magnet is applied to the human body, magnetic waves pass through the tissue and secondary currents are induced. When these currents clash with magnetic waves, they produce impacting heats on the electrons in the body cells. The impacting heats are very effective to reduce pains and swelling in the muscles, etc.

Movement of hemoglobin in blood vessels is accelerated while calcium and cholesterol deposits in blood are decreased. Even the other unwanted materials adhering to the inner side of blood vessels, which provide high blood pressure, are decreased and made to vanish. The blood is cleansed and circulation is increased. The activity of the heart eases and fatigue and pain disappear.

Functions of autonomic nerves are normalized so that the internal organs controlled by them regain their proper function.

Secretion of hormones is promoted with the result that the skin gains lustre, youth is preserved, and all ailments due to lack of hormone secretion are relieved and cured.

Blood and lymph circulations are activated and, therefore, all nutrients are easily and efficiently carried to every cell of the body. This helps in promoting the general metabolism.

Magnetic waves penetrate the skin, fatty tissue and bones, invigorating the organs. The result is greatly enhanced resistance to disease.

The magnetic flux promotes health and provides energy by eliminating disorders in, and stimulating the functions of the various systems of the body, namely the circulatory, nervous, respiratory, digestive and urinary.

The magnetic treatment works by reforming, reviving and promoting the growth of cells, rejuvenating the tissues of the body, strengthening the decayed and inactive corpuscles and increasing the number of new, sound blood corpuscles.

Magnets have exceptional curative effects on certain complaints like toothache, stiffness of shoulders and other joints, pains and swellings, cervical spondylitis, eczema, asthma as well as on chilblains, injuries and wounds.

The self-curative faculty (homeostasis) of the body is improved and strengthened which ensures all the benefits mentioned above. One feels in full vigor and can walk and work more and more without feeling tired...

NOTE: As magnets work on human metabolism mainly through the circulation of blood, which contains hemoglobin and iron, it will be relevant to state the composition of iron contained in the body. The adult human body contains 4 to 5 grams of iron and it can be traced in all parts of the body. Most of it is present in blood as a component of hemoglobin and a smaller amount remains in muscles and is called myoglobin. The function of these components is to carry oxygen from the lungs to muscles and other parts. Without iron there would be no energy, and without energy, the beating of the heart and respiration would stop. Thus, we see that iron is very essential for our life and magnetism influences iron radically and magnificently.

New Applications for the Treatment of Pain, Fatigue, and Sleep Disorders
By Robert Lang, M.D.

Magnetic therapy certainly isn't new. In fact, according to Edward A. Hacmac, D.C., it was used more than 100,000 years ago in Africa where African bloodstone (magnetite) was mined for use in potions, foods, and for topical application. Recent advances have exploited the healing power of magnets to a degree never before possible.

Before we discuss these breakthroughs in treatment, a little background is necessary. Western medicine (indeed, the western mind) has traditionally been based on the physical and mental aspects of the human body; energy was not merely not addressed, it was ridiculed. However, In 1971 when President Nixon visited China, a New York Times reporter, James Reston, developed acute appendicitis. He reported the successful use of acupuncture to relieve pain during his recovery. Overnight the west acknowledged that there was more to the human body than we could explain by our existing physical/mental model of human beings.

In fact, for most of their existence, human beings have slept and worked outdoors and were constantly exposed to the earth's magnetic field. In the Orient, as well as other parts of the world, healers have advised people to sleep with their head pointing toward the north pole in order to take advantage of the earth's magnetic field to energize the body. (Biologists have discovered that many animals instinctively sleep with their head pointed northward.) Now that we sleep on beds that contain metal springs, frames, etc., and in buildings that contain a lot of metal objects and structural components, we no longer benefit from being energized by the earth's magnetic field. Dr. Kyorchi Nakagawa and many other scientists have postulated that many people are suffering from a deficiency of magnetic energy. The symptoms include stiffness of the shoulders, back, and neck; chest pain, headache, dizziness, insomnia, constipation, fatigue, etc. Affected subjects do not respond to contemporary treatments but do have dramatic improvement after exposure to magnetic fields.

Magnets put out a powerful form of energy that can clearly affect other matter some distance away (iron filings being the most obvious example). In addition, it is known that the human body is an electromagnet by virtue of the electric charge on every living cell; anything with an electric charge has a magnetic field around it. In oriental medicine, when the body and mind are healthy, energy flows through discrete channels or meridians which are familiar to us through acupuncture. When there is a physical or mental distress, there is a block in the energy flow resulting in symptoms such as pain, swelling, etc. When the energy flow is restored with a therapeutic modality such as acupuncture, shiatsu massage, or magnetic therapy, the symptoms are relieved.

Although magnetic therapy has been around for a long time, two recent innovations have made this type of treatment more effective for pain, fatigue, and sleep disorders.

First, mattresses and mattress pads with magnets have proven to be very effective. Recent double-blind studies of patients with pain (neck, shoulders, back, and lower limbs), fatigue, and insomnia have shown that 70-85% of people using the magnetic mattresses realized an improvement in their symptoms. Patients with similar symptoms who slept on mattresses that didn't contain magnets had a modest placebo response. Of interest is that some people who slept on the mattresses with magnets noted a detoxification reaction. That is, they had a recurrence of previous symptoms from organs that had been toxic.

My personal experience is that even "healthy" people can benefit from sleeping on a magnetic mattress or mattresspad because they will note that they need one to two hours less sleep each night and have more energy. Could this be a consequence of a deficiency of exposure to the earth's magnetic field as noted above? The answer is still speculative but the results speak for themselves.

A second innovation of magnetic therapy is the result of an invention by the German physicist Horst Baermann. He discovered that by alternating concentric rings of north and south pole magnets, he could greatly increase the therapeutic effectiveness of magnets. His magnets have been tested at M.I.T., as well as other institutions around the world and have been shown to increase blood flow more effectively than ordinary bar magnets. The increased blood flow, of course, will increase the delivery of oxygen and nutrients to a diseased area as well as remove toxins that have accumulated. With these magnets, I have seen remarkable improvement in patients with pain from carpal tunnel syndrome, tendonitis, muscle strain, arthritis, low back pain, neck pain, headaches, etc. In some cases, there has been improvement when every other treatment has failed. I recently gave a magnet to a professional acupuncturist who had chronic shoulder pain which was relieved (only temporarily) by using a three inch needle on his shoulder. He experienced more effective relief with the concentric ring magnet than with any other device or medication. (Incidentally, he had tried bar magnets previously with only slight benefit).

If we look back in history it is apparent that at least 50% of what was known to be absolutely true was, in fact, false. There is now reason to believe that at least some of the disorders that we now call "functional" or psychosomatic will turn out to be problems with energy flow and/or deficiency. Based on results with magnetic mattresses and concentric magnetic pads, I believe that we will be treating many more patients with "energy medicine" in the future.

Dr. Lang is Board Certified in Internal Medicine and in Endocrinology and Metabolism. He has done research in bone diseases, nutrition, kidney stones, chronic pain, and the relationship of the mind and body in causing illness and healing. He was on the faculty of Yale Medical School for ten years. Five years ago he established Working Well International to explore new methods of healing. He has offices in New Haven and Bridgeport.

Magnetism—The Force That's Always With You
By Curt Suplee

More than 4,000 years ago, somebody made a simple discovery that forever altered the future of mankind: A kind of rock called lodestone has eerie power to attract bits of iron through some kind of invisible force.

Today, we call that phenomenon magnetism. We have learned to exploit it lavishly in generators, electric motors and hundreds of everyday devices from loudspeakers and credit cards to VCRs and TV sets......

How Magnetism Works

'The bad news is that Earth's magnetic field reverses polarity roughly every 200,000 years, but no one knows why. During the transition, the field may become very weak or disappear for awhile.'

Magnetism is one aspect of the fundamental force called electromagnetism. Electricity, which is the flow of electrons through a wire or in a beam across open space, is the other. Magnetism arises when electrically charged things move. It doesn't matter whether the charges are negative (as in electrons) or positive (as in protons). No motion, no magnetism...

Earth has a magnetic field because, deep within its core, molten metals carrying electrical charges circulate in patterns.

Earth's field also deflects charged particles, just as the field in a TV picture tube deflects moving electrons. That's good news for terrestrial life. If the planet had no magnetic field, the "solar wind"—a spray of electrons and protons blown off the sun—would strike and destroy the ozone layer, allowing Earth to be bombarded by deadly ultraviolet radiation.

Particles that make up atoms also have magnetic fields for the same reason that Earth does—they embody electrical charges in motion. For one thing, all particles spin. Also electrons travel in orbit around the nucleus of their atom. Thus all particles produce very small but measurable magnetic forces.

> 'Despite the way we usually talk, the Earth's northern hemisphere actually has a south magnetic pole. Since opposites attract, this is why the north poles of compass needles point that way.'

Actually, protons and electrons do not physically spin. But because they act as if they do, physicists have borrowed the term to describe their behavior, which otherwise is quite mysterious. Similarly, electrons do not actually orbit atoms. They exist in a cloud around the nucleus. But again, they behave as if they were circling the atom.

All atoms are miniature magnets, a result of the motion of their component parts. In most materials, atoms are oriented in different ways, so that the fields cancel each other. A few materials, such as those made of iron, cobalt and nickel, can become large-scale magnets because their atoms readily arrange themselves and their electrons so they all point the same way. That is, for example, how "natural" magnets, called lodestone, are created. As sediments containing iron-rich mineral particles are slowly deposited in layers at the bottoms of lakes and rivers, their atoms are gently tugged into alignment with the Earth's much larger field. When the mud solidifies into rock, its atoms retain that orientation, becoming permanent magnets....

How Do Magnets Let You See Inside Molecules?

Many superconducting magnets....will be used in a technique called nuclear magnetic resonance. In its most familiar form, NMR produces the magnetic resonance image (MRI) scans used in medicine. It is made possible because the magnetic properties of each element's nucleus are different.

Ordinarily, these nuclei spins are oriented at random. But when placed in a strong magnetic field, many are pulled into near-alignment with the field. Then they start revolving in a wobbling spin called precession, similar to what happens when a spinning top slows down.

The sample then is bombarded with a second, alternating magnetic field at right angles to the first. This field is switched on and off at the same rate as the spin of the hydrogen nuclei. When the second field is pulsing at exactly the right frequency, it reinforces the energy of the spinning nucleus, just as pushing a swing at precisely the right moment will make it go higher.

That condition, called "resonance," makes the nucleus tip 90 degrees or even flip over and reverse its polarity temporarily before "relaxing" back to its original alignment. And because any moving magnetic field will induce a small current in a nearby conductor, the number of tips, flips and relaxations can be measured as tiny voltages in a detector.

By using stronger magnetic fields, researchers hope to devise MRI machines two or three times more sensitive than current models. In addition, [the work is to include] determining the precise position and atomic bonds of other key biological elements such as calcium, sodium and potassium.

Tracing NMR changes in phosphorus nuclei, for example, can show how molecules of adenosine triphosphate (ATP, the energy source of life) behave in living tissue....

How Magnetism Works

MAGNETIC ORIGINS

1. Magnetism is created by atoms. It comes partly from motion of the nucleus but much more from the electrons as they fly around the nucleus.

Each electron spins, causing it to behave like a tiny bar magnet. The magnetism reaches into the surrounding space, creating "lines of force." More magnetism is created as the spinning electron moves around the nucleus.

The end result is a tiny magnet with a north and south pole and lines of force in the surrounding space.

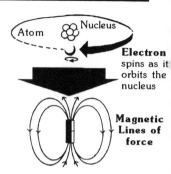

Electron spins as it orbits the nucleus

Magnetic Lines of force

MAKING METAL MAGNETIC

2. Some metals such as iron, nickel and cobalt, can be made into magnets. At first, their atoms are oriented in all directions. As a result, their magnetic fields cancel out each other. But if the metal is stroked with a magnet, its force will pull some of the atoms into alignment. The metal becomes magnetized.

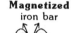

Unmagnetized iron bar

Magnetized iron bar

EARTH AS A MAGNET

3. Earth itself is a giant magnet, apparently because of electrons moving within the planet's core of iron and nickel, much as in the bar magnet. What we think of as the north pole is actually the magnetic south pole.

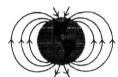

Magnetic south pole

MAGNETISM AND ELECTRICITY

4. A magnetic field also exists around wire that is conducting electricity. As the electrons flow through as electrical current, their magnetic force surrounds the wire in circles. These lines of force go around in one direction, which can be demonstrated by carrying a compass needle around a wire.

When a wire is coiled, the repeated force fields in close proximity combine to create a much stronger force through the center.

Just as electrons moving through a wire cause a magnetic field, a magnetic field moving past a wire causes a current to flow through the wire. This is the phenomenon underlying electrical generators and motors.

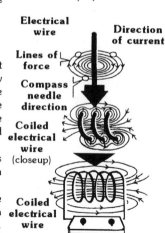

Electrical wire

Direction of current

Lines of force

Compass needle direction

Coiled electrical wire (closeup)

Coiled electrical wire

By Laura Stanton—The Washington Post

Magnetic Field Therapy: Professional and Personal Observations

By Edward Friedler, M.D.

I use magnetic products and I recommend magnetic products to my patients. I sponsored an introductory lecture on Magnetic Field Therapy to other family physicians. Is this professional heresy, or open mindedness with the interest of my patients coming first.

My formal training in Family Practice required exposure to all the traditional medical and surgical specialties. A family physician must have a wide array of management options for his or her patients. In spite of years of training and clinical experience, it is unfortunately not unusual for my "bag of tricks" to be unsatisfactory or empty! Because it is anathema for me to tell patients "There is nothing more I can do for you," I have referred some to chiropractors and not discouraged others seeking help through other "alternative" providers. And now, I am one too!

I use magnetic products for a variety of ailments. Because I see people in the setting of a medical office, there is an expectation that *any* treatment is recommended after a working diagnosis is made. In other words, I listen to and examine my patients and get appropriate lab information and x-rays first. Once the data is collected and considered and a working diagnosis made, I then organized a discussion on treatment options. For the person complaining of fatigue, I treat anemia with iron and vitamins, not a magnet. For a person with achy legs and low potassium, I treat with potassium, not a magnet. Yet there are times when iron, potassium, aspirin, or a narcotic pain pill are not the appropriate remidies, or are not enough. In these cases, I encourage my patients to try a magnet. Let me share some success stories.

Cancer. Dr. F was diagnosed with cancer at age 41. After three months of chemotherapy, he decided that because the track record for chemotherapy was poor, it would be *crazy* to not add other modalities to his own treatment. Since his oncologist was concerned with chemotherapy dosing, and didn't know about other treatments, Dr. F on his own added Magnetic Field Therapy, via a mattress pad, chair pads in the office and home, and a large magnet worn agains the lower spine. (Dr. F added other "modalities" over the next few months.) He experienced fewer negative side effects of chemotherapy, to the surprise of his oncologist. He lived, and still lives to tell about it, I am happy to say, because Dr. F is me!

Arthritis. I remember Mrs. R whose knee joint had no cartilage. No medicine prescribed by me or other doctors had helped her. I taped a small magnet to her knee after a physical exam, and left the room while she got dressed. When I came back to minutes later, she was bending her knee in disbelief; it didn't hurt. The arthritis wasn't gone, but the severe pain was.

> 'I tell my patients about magnets, and I show them the *Magnetic Field Therapy Handbook* as a guide to usage. I have not had anyone say, "No thanks, I would rather suffer."'

Fractured rib. Mr. E had fallen and broken a rib; his oncologist had given him Percocet for pain. He came in to see me, saying the rib still hurt, and the drug made him feel bad. I advised him to place a magnet where the pain was causing him discomfort. He later told me the diminishment of pain was "instantaneous." The rib was still broken, but he was able to discontinue the Percocet. When he broke another rib two months later, he used a magnet first.

Brown recluse spider bite. Mr. W was bitten by a brown recluse spider. He had a one inch ulcer on his lower leg that was not healing. It hurt, too. We taped a magnet over the ulcer. The pain was less and it began to heal up quickly. The magnet, while he used it decreased the pain.

Swollen eye. A boy had been hit in the face by a baseball. His eyelids were swollen. He had already used ice. I gave him a mini magnet and told him to use it where the sting occured. The swelling was gone the next day. I was surprised.

Shoulder pain. Dr. Q was experiencing a nagging pain in her shoulder for more than three months. She attended the lecture on Magnetic Field Therapy. During this event she held a magnet to her shoulder. The next morning, her shoulder was normal and the pain was gone. My own theory is she used the magnet on her own. (At that same meeting, another doctor used a magnet on a painful knee, which had been through many drugs and physical therapy. The next day, she came to my office for a second magnet, because it was helping her so much.)

Tiredness. When all the test are normal, doctors often diagnose depression for tired people. Some respond to antidepressant treatment. For Ms. E, magnetic shoe inserts worked. She even returned to her karate class.

As a physician I prefer to understand as fully as possible the workings and applications of Magnetic Field Therapy. I study this in my own practice. I tell my patients about magnets, and I show them the *Magnetic Field Therapy Handbook* as a guide to usage. I have not had anyone say, "No thanks, I would rather suffer." I am grateful to have Magnetic Field Therapy as a positive intervention for helping the patients in my medical practice.

Why Magnetic Therapy Works
By Leane E. Roffey

After many months of research with clients, it appears that the application of permanent magnetic field therapy in conjunction with various forms of bodywork can induce rapid positive changes in the body. These changes include: reducing symptoms of pain, especially in the back and the extremities; enhancing tissue release during anatriptic work; and modifying psychosomatic behavioral conditions, such as reducing anxiety.

This article discusses why exposing a client to a permanent magnetic field, such as on a magnetic mat or a locally placed magnetic pad, seems to facilitate and enhance the effects of anatriptic work. To find the answers, we must first look at the connective tissue system and examine what properties it has biomechanically and electrically, and then relate the mechanisms to what we know about biomagnetics. The search to understand this has led me through a morass of papers, books and documents, but the picture which finally emerged made it all worthwhile. Hopefully, the following explanation will serve as an introduction for practitioners of the anatriptic arts to encourage the use of permanent magnetic tools that provide uniform magnetic fields, especially mats and magnets, just as they would use other mechanical devices.

In order to understand the how and why of magnetic therapy, it is necessary to briefly review the "electronic nature" of the connective tissue system, especially the fascia, for in its structure and priorities lies the very basis for the mechanism of a magnetic effect on tissue. We will examine first the whole system, then the cells and finally the process of molecular ionic exchange to set the stage for the biomagnetic connection.

Connective tissue provides a continuous medium throughout the body. It is a composite material, made up of collagen fibers embedded in a gel-like ground substance, called the Extra Cellular Matrix (ECM). These collagen fibers are arranged in an ordered, crystalline array. Like other crystals, connective tissue is piezoelectric. That is, it generates electric fields when compressed or stretched. Since collagen is a semiconductor, the connective tissue forms an "integrated electronic network" in the human body, allowing all parts of the organism to communicate.

Fascia are sheets of connective tissue. The myofascia, for example, are collagenous fascial sheets which cover muscles and fibers. Fascia are slightly mobile and continuous from head to toe, and is found in and around all of the somatic and visceral structures of the human body. As a membrane, it is tough, thick and durable. The collagenous fibers, as an example, have tensile strength up to 2,000 pounds per square inch.

In his book, *Craniosacral Therapy*, Dr. John Upledger points out that fascia is largely oriented in a longitudinal direction and is free to glide on the order of millimeters when the body musculature is relaxed. Transverse layers of fascia and connective tissue form the diaphragms we are all familiar with—thoracic, respiratory, pelvic floor. You can literally travel from any part of the body to any other part via the fascia.

Upledger further states that, with this idea in mind, it is apparent that any loss of mobility of this tissue in a specific area can be used as a guide to help locate a disease or malfunction which has caused that lack of mobility. This is an important realization because it means that, if the fascia is a semiconductive "electronic network," the strain patterns caused by trauma, whether physical or emotional, are communicated to adjacent structures in the body. Adjacent myofascial structures may be "glued" to each other, and thickening and foreshortening of tissue may result. The tensional force is transferrable, and the body may compensate for the injury systemically. This compensation provides a traceable "road map" directly back to the area which initially malfunctioned.

A special type of fascial tissue is the soft tissue called the meningeal membrane, or meninges, which envelops the brain and spinal cord. There are three meningeal layers, the dura mater, the arachnoid membrane and the pia mater. The dura mater is the external layer of the three. It is a tough, relatively inelastic connective tissue which is fused with the internal aspect of the skull. It forms vertical sheets, the falces cerebri and cerebelli, which separate the hemispheres of the cerebrum and the cerebellum respectively. It also forms the relatively horizontal sheets, the tentorium cerebelli, bilaterally, which separate the cerebrum from the cerebellum. It is the dura mater which contains the cerebrospinal fluid.

The arachnoid membrane is thin and delicate. It is separated from the dura and the pia mater by the subdural and subarachnoid spaces, which are filled with fluid. The pia mater is the highly vascularized, delicate internal layer of the meningeal membrane. It follows all of the convolutions of the brain and spinal cord and supplies blood.

The meninges have continuity with the fascias of the body through a very complicated network of connective tissue, which wraps around all organs, muscles and other structures. The loss of mobility in a specific area can be used as a starting point to trace back the strain patterns not only through the limbs and torso but through the meninges to the inner dural structures around the brain itself. The sources of somato-emotional dysfun-ctions may be traceable to these strain patterns in the cranium.

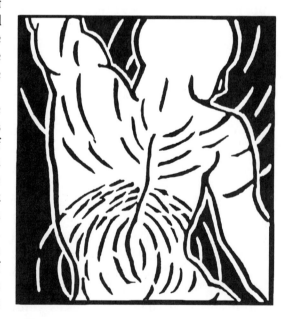

From the standpoint of physics the tensional force of the fascia becomes a key component in the electronic network communication throughout the body. All movement of the body as a whole or of the smallest of its parts is created by tensions carried through the connective tissue fabric whether natural or unnatural. Vectors or lines of tensional force become increasingly important to analyze when working on a client.

The body has a moveable skeleton and a system of soft parts that gives it form but so does each cell. Recent electron microscopic research shows that each cell has its own mini-myofascial system made up of a skeleton of tubules interconnected with a somewhat mobile fibrous ground substance. There are other substances called glycoproteins that extend across the cell membrane. They are connected to the filamentous network within the cell.

Outside the cell these glycoproteins form branching structures with charged groups (actually sialic acid) at the ends of the branches. These in turn are joined by means of ionic calcium bridges to the negatively charged ends of the molecules comprising the extracellular matrix. An additional set of proteins, called fibronectins, binds the cell surface to extracellular collagenous fibers. These, along with the gel of the connective tissue, ultimately interconnect with the larger fiber arrays of the myofascial system, including tendons, muscles and bones.

Molecularly, muscle and connective tissue are not pure protein crystals because water and ions are also present. The water molecules and ions are not randomly dispersed but are attracted to the protein structure in a regular repeating pattern. This is why connective tissue is a highly ordered piezoelectric system. When compressed, piezoelectric crystals produce weak electric fields. Therefore, every movement of the body which implies even the slightest myofascial involvement generates weak electric fields. In addition electric fields can also occur as a consequence of nerve conduction and the activation of muscle contraction. Even gland secretion can give rise to electric fields. These fields spread throughout the tissue, providing signals that inform cells of movements, loads or other activity. The cells in turn use this information to adjust their activities in maintaining and nourishing the surrounding tissues.

Electrophysiologically, then, this "electronic network" is transmitted through the tissue and propagated through surrounding membranes by the regenerative property inherent in the action potentials of the cells themselves. These action potentials are phenomena associated with the electrical impulses generated when neuron clusters of excitable nerve tissues are stimulated, i.e., during synaptic transmission.

It is not yet completely known how all synapses convey impulses. Transmission of the weak electrical field may be caused by chemical transmitters or by electrical conduction across low-resistance pathways. Nerves that convey excitatory impulses make up the sympathetic nervous system. The viscera are the province of the parasympathetic nervous system. Together they comprise the autonomic nervous system. Half the sympathetic nervous system, called the vasomotor system, regulates the rate and flow of blood through the body. The remainder innervates all the soft tissue such as the skin, muscles, tendons, ligaments and fascial tissue.

It is next important to understand exactly how the piezoelectric signal gets from a connective tissue fiber under stress to a nearby fibroblast cell, and then to the cell nucleus to regulate protein synthesis. Certainly ionic exchange and action potential between the cells may be part of the answer, but, intuitively, a literal "quantum" leap on the subatomic level is more likely to be at the root of why this function occurs.

Bioelectric signals automatically produce biomagnetic fields. Protein systems seem to be natural continuous energy systems. Organic systems have semiconductor characteristics. Protons as well as electrons are highly dependent on the amount of hydration present. The presence of hydrogen ions and the degree to which the weak electrical signals are "organized" may be an important mechanism. What is the possible significance of this for higher levels of structure such as the fascia? Does exposure to a permanent compatible weak magnetic field somehow make the dispersion of charge and/or energy more efficient or better organize the signals in the electronic network?

Let us examine the case of tissue which is glued and/or under tension to see if an answer becomes obvious. When an orthopedic type injury occurs, either induced by velocity injuries or extreme tension, cells are stimulated to generate additional connective tissue fibers which bind and protect the area of injury. Normally these fibers later would be removed and replaced with healthy tissue at some rate by the natural processes the body uses. Often, however, the rate of assembly exceeds the rate of removal and the fibers build up. As a result of this buildup on the cellular level, the ground substance of the extracellular matrix solidifies. The fascia thickens and shortens, and there is a side-effect of dehydration. Water is driven out of the ground substance. The extracellular matrix loses much of its electrical conductivity as a result.

Metabolic wastes then begin to accumulate, resulting in conditions of fatigue. Most important, there is a distinct loss of electrical activity through the tissue. The sodium/potassium ion pump is disturbed, which interferes with nerve impulse conduction through unmyelinated fibers. A condition known as paresthesia results. Nerve endings become irritated, causing pain, numbness, pressure and/or hot and cold sensations. Because of the weak electrical conductive nature of the fascial tissue, sometimes symptoms may occur far from the site of the injury. Immobilization and stiffness are also side effects, and collagenous tissue may build up within and across the joint spaces.

The body employs compensatory mechanisms, sacrificing function to safeguard structural integrity. From a biomechanical standpoint, the fascial planes communicate localized strain throughout the entire body, and a spiraling pattern of contraction occurs dispersing the force of the strain throughout the surrounding tissue. Proprioceptive memory adapts to the shortened muscle or injured disk as "normal."

Excessive neurological activity also occurs in the ligaments and the tendinous attachments of the muscle. Further, this tension is communicated to the brain through the dura, which is pulled or compressed in the direction of the strain. The "strain lines" are communicated via the "electronic network" up the dura and are reflected in the inner cranial structures, particularly the falx cerebri. The interesting thing about this entire process is that when the injury reaches this stage, there is no difference to the client psychosomatically between the injury and the psychological effect of the injury. The tension becomes "locked" in the client's psychosomatic structure, and becomes part of their emotional framework.

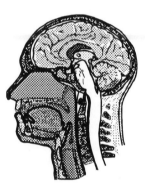

The stress stimuli continue to increase, since the system is stymied at this point, so the tone of the sympathetic nervous system rises. The parasympathetic nervous system must also rise in tone to counteract the sympathetic system effect. Finally, a point is reached in which the parasympathetic system cannot cope with or effectively counteract the increased energy of the sympathetic system. The autonomic nervous system loses its flexibility, and functional disease results. The client develops disease, either psychosomatic or actual, and is generally driven to seek help, either physical or mental to obviate the stress and pain they feel.

Enter the anatriptic practitioner, who uses a variety of techniques to begin to effect change in the client. If a practitioner moves or asks for movement of the affected tissue into its correct anatomical position through slow, micro-like motions, spikes occur in the electrical activity of the cells, and arouse sympathetic nervous system response in surrounding body areas.

Current is generated by a piezoelectric-like effect through the fascial planes during anatriptic practice which can significantly influence metabolism and the cellular activity. As the practitioner applies pressure to the skin and the tissues with intent, the electrical cellular activity begins to increase. Subsequent connective tissue manipulation results in re-hydration, increased electrical conductivity, increased blood supply, and re-education of collagen fiber thickening. The extracellular matrix goes from a gel state to a more liquid state, toxins are flushed, and the gel reforms in a healthier, more organized manner.

In addition, a greater efficiency of a biomechanical phenomenon is achieved through anatriptic practices such as neuromuscular massage, craniosacral balancing, energy work, and especially myofascial release technique.

Mobility can be restored and joints made to move more freely. The balancing of centers of mass with respect to gravity is even possible through techniques such as Rolfing and deep myofascial work. Upledger indicates, for example, one of the beneficial effects of many of the therapeutic techniques he uses via the craniosacral system is the restoration of autonomic flexibility. Because the autonomic nervous system plays such a large role in the homeostatic activity of the body, when autonomic flexibility is restored, many homeostatic mechanisms are made more effective.

At this point, it is useful to examine the craniosacral system in more detail. Upledger has put forth a "pressurestat" model to explain the rhythmic rise and fall of fluid pressure in this system. The pressure causes the rhythmic changes in the boundaries of the semihydraulic system comprised of the meninges, cranium, spine and sacrum. He hypothesizes that the presence of certain structures in the system supports a mechanism whereby the reproduction of cerebrospinal fluid is under homeostatic control. He suggests that it is a "pressurestat" mechanism which causes the ventricular system of the brain to dilate and contract in a rhythmic fashion. Within the four ventricles of the brain the cerebrospinal fluid is produced.

The force of pressure is a type of stress which is exerted per unit area. Cranial fluid exerts slight wave-like pressure on the dural membranes which form the boundary of the cerebrospinal fluid hydraulic system. At any given time, within the dura, there is about one half cup of cerebrospinal fluid circulating in the system. The fact that this is a semi-closed hydraulic system means there is the introduction and re-absorption of cerebrospinal fluid. Hydraulically, when you have fluid pressure in the brain because of the introduction of cerebrospinal fluid, a swelling occurs which presses outward against the cranial bones.

The cranium has sutures which stretch slightly. When they reach an end point of movement, they hit stretch receptors. The receptors send a signal back to stop fluid production. When the production of the cerebrospinal fluid is stopped, a mechanism called the arachnoid granulations takes out the spent fluid and puts it back into venous drainage, causing the head to shrink back. At the end point of contraction, pressure receptors are activated which signal the choroid plexus (the mechanism in the ventricular structure which filters the fluid) to resume fluid production. The entire head, meninges and brain have very slight movement. This system has very precise motility, which is the rhythmic response in the soft tissue to an intrinsic pulse.

We particularly want to consider the biomagnetic composition of the tissue in this semi-hydraulic system. In addition to electrical and biomechanical forces, there are also neuromagnetic phenomena present in the body tissue, especially in the meningeal membrane and throughout the brain tissue. These phenomena are also traceable throughout the body, and, in the opinion of this researcher, it is the fascial, principally the meningeal, tissue which provides the primary channel through which biomagnetic current is transmitted throughout the body. The connective tissue system is actually a delicately-tuned and extremely sensitive detector, amplifier and processor of electromagnetic signals.

As for the origin of these neuromagnetic field phenomena, during excitatory signal transmission from one neuron to another (for a period of 10-100 milliseconds) a current in the 10-100 pico Ampere range flows along a dendrite for a distance of a few tenths of a millimeter. This electrical flow is like that from a battery and can be considered the primary or source current. At the same time, return currents flow in the surrounding medium (typically fascial tissue), completing the current path.

It can be seen that thousands of aligned neurons would act in synchronicity to produce a rather large total primary current on the order of microamperes. This current produces a magnetic field in the range of 500-5,000 pico gauss, which can be detected outside the head. An example may be represented by a dipole, the strength of which would be the product of the primary current amplitude and path length. However, if the activity is distributed over a larger area, several dipoles or a distributed source model would be required to represent the field.

An opportunity to non-invasively record and analyze neural events with millisecond resolution arises in the field of Magnetoencephalography (MEG). This technique uses the ultrasensitive Superconducting Quantum Interference Devices (SQUID Magnetometers) as a study tool. Work done by Ilmoneimi at the Helsinki University of Technology using a 24-channel SQUID Magnetometer has established that there is a rapidly changing magnetic field pattern over the occipital head, produced by neuronal currents in the brain.

Ilmoneimi plans work in the near future with an improved device having an array of over 100 channels, offering the possibility of studying complex phenomena involving several distinct cerebral areas at one time and possibly to define a distributed source model for neural activity.

Other SQUID magnetometer studies (Kirschvink et al.) which involved sampling and extraction of brain tissue revealed two distinct types of magnetic crystals within brain cells. Most importantly the human brain tissue has the unmistakable signature of the ferromagnetic mineral magnetite. It is well known that ferromagnetic materials are those that interact strongly with a magnetic field.

Ferromagnetic materials are contrasted with diamagnetic materials that are weakly repelled by magnetic fields, such as water and most fatty substances, and paramagnetic materials that are weakly attracted by magnetic fields like some of the iron in the hemoglobin molecule which carries oxygen in the blood, as well as oxygen itself.

All areas of the brain have been found to have significant levels of magnetite—about four nanograms of magnetite per gram of brain tissue—but the highest levels were associated with the meninges, which had about 70 nanograms of magnetite per gram of tissue. Kirschvink notes that at 70 nanograms per gram, magnetite makes up only a small fraction of the iron in brain tissue. However, even if only one cell in a million contains it, this small fraction could have a large effect when exposed to magnetic fields!

Therefore, a permanent magnetic field could be expected to have an effect, possibly on the quantum level, in all electrically conductive tissue in the body. This is why weak electrical signals released through anatriptic work in the presence of such a magnetic field move rapidly throughout the tissue. The presence of a harmonic magnetic field acts to support the transmission of neuromagnetic current throughout the body, which in turn augments and supports electrical signal release occurring in the tissues. It is as if placing the body in a uniform magnetic field induces electrical current release in a orderly and systematic fashion, with the cranial rhythm acting as a driving mechanism.

In physics, the field of magnetohydrodynamics is concerned with the study of the dynamics or motion of an electrically conducting fluid interacting with a magnetic field. Up until this time, this science has been primarily concerned with properties of ionized gases and liquid metals. When the extracellular matrix undergoes its gel-to-sol-to-gel reorganization during anatriptic work, it is behaving as if it were an electrically conducting medium, a "viscoplastic" substance which rehydrates under pressure and reforms when the pressure is released.

In magnetohydrodynamics there is a dimensionless number, symbolized by N, known as a magnetic force parameter. It contains terms of magnetic permeability, magnetic field strength, electrical conductivity, a characteristic length, mass density and fluid velocity.

In parallel, fascial tissue has magnetic permeability, magnetic field strength, electrical conductivity, and mass density. There is a fluid velocity inherent in the tissue which, although not yet exactly defined, apparently can be affected by both pressure and magnetic field strength. Typical anatriptic practices induce electrical release, using pressure and/or velocity.

'The connective tissue system is actually a delicately-tuned and extremely sensitive detector, amplifier and processor of electromagnetic signals.'

All the elements are present to begin to define a simple model of the magnetic force parameter for the fascial tissue. Elements of the fascia, especially the extracellular matrix, may be a type of "magnetofluid," whose flow properties become viscoplastic when modulated by a magnetic field and may be subject to laws of magnetohydrodynamic stability.

It is assumed that some kind of magnetic resonance is at work to explain the useful phenomena observed and discussed above. This kind of resonance in which the presence of a magnetic field can influence, enhance and facilitate some of the physical and chemical change processes, is a phenomenon exhibited by the magnetic spin systems of certain atoms. Spin systems absorb energy at specific frequencies when subjected to magnetic fields alternating at frequencies which are synchronistic with natural system frequencies.

Permanent magnetism affects both hydrogen-ion exchange and acid-alkali balance in paramagnetic substances containing oxygen. These activities occur in the human metabolic system, so perhaps magnetic resonance is an important factor to be considered in determining which natural field strengths provide the best exposure for the human system....

In this paper it has been shown that the fascial tissue (particularly the meninges) is magnetic, fluidic and possesses weak electrical properties. It is also pressure sensitive. These properties—weak electrical signals released through anatriptic work, especially in the presence of a permanent magnetic field of appropriate strength—are compatible and synergistic. The presence of the magnetic field acts as a medium for the transmission of neuromagnetic current throughout the fascial tissue of the body which augments and enhances the release of neuroelectrical signals.

It is conceivable, therefore, using the pressurestat craniosacral model as the pump, that magnetohydrodynamic wave phenomena can occur throughout the entire fascial system of the body, and that this phenomena may be a two-way path. Manipulating the fascia can affect the balance of the craniosacral system, and craniosacral balancing affects the fascia.

From a physics standpoint, theory suggests that the low pressurestat model of the craniosacral system provides a source of subtle magnetohydrodynamic waves, resulting in wave-like motion of electric current through the semi-fluidic fascial tissue and other more fluidic systems of the body. The presence of an external magnetic field can be expected to influence this process significantly.

Leane Rofey is a bioengineer and systems analyst, and is listed in Who's Who in the World and Who's Who in Science and Engineering. She also operates a small research and development firm called Neuro Magnetic Systems.

In order to avoid unnecessary injury to your horse and to obtain the maximum benefit from the unique features of magnet therapy the following suggestions and recommendations are offered:

1. Consult with your vet to determine whether magnet therapy is an appropriate therapy for the specific injury.

2. Do not place a [magnetic pad] on an area that has had paint or liniment on it. The petrochemical base of many preparations will tend to degrade the polyethylene matrix of the pads. Wash all areas of application very thoroughly with soap and water and leave uncovered for approximately 24 hours prior to the application of the magnetic pads.

3. The pads should be placed as close to the skin as possible without causing excessive pressure to, or aggravation of, the condition being treated. It is also recommended the area be checked to make sure it is thoroughly dry and has remained clean.

4. Placement:

Leg. The large pad ("Flex") should be placed on the back of the canon with the wider end down and with the soft cotton side facing the leg. Wrap the leg as usual with regular leg wrapping bandages to secure the pad (the hook style material on the back of the pad will serve to anchor the pad within the bandage).

For use on the front of the canon, place the pad on the shin with the wide end up and cotton side also facing the leg, and affix in a similar manner as the back.

NOTE: Another, stronger, type of application using several strip- or band-type pads can be substituted for any of the applications mentioned here and is simplified through the use of a soft cotton cloth cover specifically designed for the purpose. This cover makes it possible to target 1, 2 or 3 separate magnets to specific areas and also select identical types (strip, band, mini or card) or intermix them depending upon the desired effect.

Forte Circle. Use a magnetic pad of the appropriate size and shape. Place a small piece of hook-style material on the surface opposite the soft cotton side to help keep the pad from shifting inside the wrapping (see "Note" above for possible alternative). For some very difficult to bandage areas, tape will most likely be the best and only alternative. Should this prove to be the case, we advise *against* using a tape with limited flexibility or strong adhesive qualities as it may cause damage to the magnet or your patient.

Pastern and Splint. The pads are placed on the intended area and wrapped as advised in the previous applications.

5. Once applied, a pad should remain in place for at least 4-6 hours, increasing by two hour intervals to a maximum length of application of approximately 20 hours per day. This gradual increase provides an opportunity for accurate assessment of the effect the application is having upon the condition being treated. If the area begins to swell it could be a sign that the modality was begun too early and should be discontinued. The area should be completely cooled down and reevaluated before beginning again after the swelling has begun to recede.

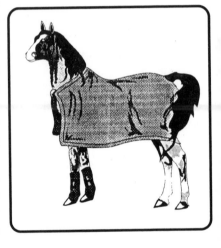

6. A recommended modality for use of the leg pads is to apply them in the morning during the normal routine, remove before the evening feed, then reapply when the legs are done up for the evening. The pads remain in place until morning, when they are removed again for a short time before starting the routine again. This routine will allow two opportunities per day for examination of the effectiveness of the therapy, and will also allow you to observe any signs of, and take corrective action for, pressure or friction sensitivity.

7. When applying any pads be careful not to place them too close to joints as the continuous flexing and torquing in this area will

eventually cause a breakdown in the material the pad is made from. Cracking, however, will not decrease the effectiveness of the pad— the pads may even be cut in half without decreasing their strength or effectiveness, and can only be destroyed by extreme heat (melting), degaussing (requires an industrial-strength electromagnet) or chemical contamination as mentioned earlier. Should your pad suffer damage in the form of cracking, simply use a strong strapping tape (duct tape is a good choice) on the back to restore its integrity. It is well to keep this adaptability of the pads in mind should you run into any special or difficult treatment requirements.

8. The degree of severity of the injury is the determining factor as to length of treatment. Naturally, a severe tendonitis will take longer to heal than a slight sprain. Please work with your vet to determine the appropriate treatment time. Most injuries will begin to exhibit signs of dramatic change within a few days.

9. After the injury has healed, it is recommended that a regular routine of application be maintained as a preventive measure. By increasing the circulation to areas being placed, or about to be placed under stress, the chances for an injury occurring are greatly reduced. IMPORTANT: It should be remembered that certain injuries to the foreleg are sometimes incorrectly assumed to be healed when the lameness has subsided. This is a very dangerous assumption as it has been found in many cases that signs of lameness do not correlate well with the extent of the injury. Caution should be exercised against returning a horse to its normal routine prematurely when it has suffered this type of injury.

10. The pads should not be used while exercising or bathing the horse. If the pads were left on during a workout, the horse could suffer further injury due to the tremendous buildup of heat in the area. While water will not damage the magnetic material itself, the cotton facing will deteriorate more rapidly under these conditions. When the cotton face becomes worn or soiled to the point that it cannot be restored by washing in a mild soap and water solution, simply peel it off and replace it with a similar material (adhesive-

backed moleskin found in the Dr. Scholl's human foot care section of your local drug store or grocery makes a great substitute).

Cautions:

Do Not Apply Magnetic Type Pads...

. . . If the horse has an active untreated infection
. . . To an area with an acute injury—cool thoroughly
. . . To a hematoma less than three days old
. . . On or near open wounds
. . . When you would normally use ice
. . . While exercising or bathing the horse
. . . Without consulting your veterinarian

Also of interest for the horse owner in the area of useful magnetic products, it has been found that the *seat cushion* or the *horse blanket* is highly appreciated when placed on the back after a long day under a saddle.

You may discover many other worthwhile applications and uses for these amazing new products and devices yourself—like the discovery that your cat or dog has developed a very strong attraction for sleeping on your bed since you got the new magnetic mattress.

Historical Perspectives

Today there is a re-awakening to the use of magnetism in the field of therapeutics. Through innovative design and revolutionary applications, biomagnetism is finding an ever-increasing niche in the health care fields of many countries throughout the world. To fully understand this phenomenon and the potential it has in our world today, it is helpful to look at some historical applications and facts about magnetism.

For thousands of years, mankind has utilized the beneficial powers of magnetism, knowing little about the specific reasons it worked or effects it created, but realizing only that curative results could be achieved.

The oldest known usages of magnetic powers is traced to Africa, where an African bloodstone (magnetite) mine more than 100,000 years old has been found. The magnetite was ground up and used in potions, food, and topical applications.

In ancient Greece, Aristotle was the first person in recorded history to speak of the therapeutic properties of the natural magnets of his time. Nevertheless, most of the ancient civilizations, including the Hebrews, Arabs, Indians, Egyptians and Chinese, used magnets for healing.

It is recorded that around 200 B.C., the Greek physician Galen found that pain from many different types of illness could be relieved by applying natural magnets.

In the first century, the Chinese began documenting effects on health and disease related to variations in the Earth's magnetic field, using very sensitive compasses to monitor those variations.

Around 1000 A.D. a Persian physician documented the use of magnets to relieve disorders such as gout and muscle spasms.

In the 1600's an English physician named Gilbert wrote of magnetism, and in the 1700's another physician named

Mesmer wrote a dissertation on magnetism that has proven to be a foundation for magnetic healing in the Western culture. Dr. Mesmer's name became synonymous with magnetism, but in a negative fashion. He was ridiculed for his advanced discoveries and his abilities to use magnetism for good. It was called "mesmerism," scoffed at as unscientific and unreliable and was deemed an unworthy practice or "Charlatanism."

Despite the increasing ridicule, other studies were performed, including the first in-depth study of the history of magnetic treatment of diseases undertaken in 1777 by France's Royal Society of Medicine. Other studies included reports by Eydam in 1843, Charot and Renard in 1878, Mueller in 1879, Benedict and Drozdov in 1879, Benedict in 1885 and Quinan in 1886.

Negative studies on magnetic therapy were forthcoming, one by Peterson and Kennelly of the influential Edison Laboratory, and another by Rosenberg, who stated in 1928 that "We must admit that until now no basis for acknowledging the effect of a constant magnetic field has been obtained." This appears to have become the established theory in western countries.

Regardless, future research and development were soon to become monumental in re-awakening the interest in biomagnetism. Beginning in the 1930's, researchers such as Davis in 1936 and Hansen in 1938 began to write of their investigations and experiments using magnetism. Hansen reported that subjective complaints were being relieved by the application of magnetism, such as in sciatica, low back pain, and joint pains....

By 1958, much work was being done in Japan, and by 1959 published reports were beginning to appear from Nakagawa, Tomizuka, and Takeyama. At that time, several medical Congresses on "Magnetism and Living Bodies" were presented and followed by three Conferences on "Magnetic Fields and Living Bodies" from 1974-1976.

Today, much continuing scientific research in France, Russia, England, Canada, India, China, Japan and the United States is providing invaluable data on how magnetic fields affect the nervous and circulatory systems, as well as every living cell, whether animal, human, or plant.

Through the use of ultra-sensitive measuring devices now available, the human body, in fact all life, is found to be electrical in nature and therefore is influenced by and responds to minute magnetic/electrical changes.

Nakagawa has reported on the existence of a group of symptomatic conditions that respond favorably to an introduction of a magnetic field, when all else has failed. He calls this group of health problems a "Magnetic Deficiency Syndrome" and documents much research in Japan on the use of magnetotherapeutic devices such as magnetic bracelets, necklaces, rings, and mattresses to treat this Syndrome.

At Massachusetts Institute of Technology, a prestigious laboratory has been established to study and document advances in magnetic field therapy and the United States Government has recently (1990) begun funding new research at Florida State University.

All these studies into the diagnostic and therapeutic benefits of magnetism promise to create a new age for an energy not totally understood yet destined to play a major role in the health care of the future.

Applications of Biomagnetism

It should be made clear that magnets themselves do not heal anything—they only stimulate the body to heal itself. Magnetism is a wholly natural event. It is neither magic nor medicine. It merely allows body cells to exist at their best level.

In recent years developments in healing through electrical and magnetic therapies have increased exponentially. In the treatment of sprains, strains, broken bones, burns and cuts, not only does magnetic field therapy aid in the recovery but it allows these conditions to heal better, more quickly, and with less scar tissue and better symmetry. In injuries, magnetic treatment has been shown to decrease healing time by half or more.

In the treatment of chronic conditions such as some forms of arthritis, degenerative joint conditions, diabetic ulcers and cancer, magnetic field therapy has shown dramatic results in aiding the reduction or reversal of the condition.

At Columbia University's Orthopedic Hospital of the Presbyterian Medical Center in New York City, Dr. Andrew Bassett, one of America's most noted researchers in magnetic and electric therapies, has achieved dramatic results using electric therapy for hip joint injuries or breaks. He has used electrically induced magnetic fields to cause regrowth of tissue, nerve, bone, and blood supply. An FDA evaluation of his work showed that approximately 85% of these hip injury patients would have needed hip replacement without the therapy.

A Reader's Digest article in October, 1982, titled "Biomagnetism: An Awesome Force in Our Lives," quoted Dr. Bassett as predicting "Electricity will become as ubiquitous in medical practice as surgery or drugs are; in many instances it will replace them."

Dr. Robert O. Becker has written extensively in his books, *The Body Electric* and *Cross Currents*, about the future usage of magnetic and electrical therapy, predicting discoveries and advancements that today would only be considered impossible or miraculous.

Doctors in both Europe and the United States are obtaining results using electromagnetic fields to treat damage ranging from decubitus ulcers to severe burns. Soft tissue injuries are responding as well as those of bone and joint. In the Soviet Union, doctors regularly use magnets to speed wound healing after surgery and to strengthen and mend bones.

Some researchers, such as Nordenstrom and Wollin have reported using super-magnets and electrical therapies to successfully treat lung and breast cancers.

An American dentist, Dr. Jack Prince, has successfully used magnets on acupuncture points to reduce bleeding, gagging and pain sensitivity. Dr. Prince found that magnets could bring immediate relief of chronic pain from jaw dislocations as well as from TMJ syndrome, headaches, and teeth grinding.

One of the leading new diagnostic methods used in modern medicine is the MRI (Magnetic Resonance Imaging). This system of visualizing soft and hard tissues within the body, without invasive techniques or x-rays, has quickly surpassed the capabilities of CAT Scans and is used to look for potential damage to injured joints or presence of abnormalities, prior to exploratory surgery. Among the other leading edge instruments and tools related to the body's biomagnetic field and being used in modern hospitals and laboratories are:

• SQUID (Superconducting Quantum Interference Device) which can detect minute changes in biomagnetic fields around body organs and thus diagnose disease;

• MEGS or magnetoencephalograms, similar to EEG;

• MKG or magnetocardiogram, similar to EKG;

• BioMagnetic Pulsar, used in more than 1000 hospitals, colleges and health care offices to administer pulsed magnetic field therapy to relieve pain, stiffness, sore throats, colds, arthritis and other problems.

In Japan, a number of licensed manufacturers of medical devices are producing magnetotherapeutic devices. One such system utilizes the placement of permanent magnets into mattresses and pillows, allowing the user to receive their therapy regularly and simply, as they sleep. It is a unique concept that gives the user maximum exposure without taking away from normal daily activity time.

Although science cannot yet fully explain what takes place when the body is placed within such a magnetic sleep system, kinesiology (muscle strength) testing shows each acupuncture meridian in the body is functioning in harmony within fifteen minutes. It logically follows that the longer a body remains in this environment, the more quickly it can balance itself.

Another effect of a magnetic field that is well documented and supported by the laws of physics is the enhancement of blood circulation and lymphatic drainage. Mattress users report increased warmth in the extremities during their sleep and also report decreased muscle and joint pain.

The circulatory effect is documented in Faraday's Law and the Hall Effect, two long accepted laws of physics that explain the principles by which the action of the magnetic polarities create ionic currents and patterns, which in turn increase the diameter of the blood vessels and ease the movement of the blood through those vessels.

Interesting and Alarming Facts on Magnetism

Variations in the earth's magnetic field are important to all the living beings on the planet. Scientists are aware that this field is in constant flux as it is influenced by solar winds, shifts in the earth's core, and the presence of ferromagnetic substances in the earth's crust.

Current research shows that the earth's field periodically waxes and wanes, and even reverses itself entirely. Though the reasons for this are not known, geological evidence indicates that the strength of the field gradually grows weaker, reaches a minimum or disappears entirely, and then builds again the opposite direction, resulting in a reversal of the north and south magnetic poles. Scientists estimate that such reversals occur about every one-half to one million years. The most recent reversal took place about 700,000 years ago.

Other scientists have documented that earth's magnetic field has degraded about 50% over the last 500-1000 years, with a full 5% decline being recorded in the past 100 years. Calculations are that if this degradation continues at its present rate, there will not be a sufficient magnetic field to support life within 1500 years.

Interestingly, certain locales on Earth have inexplicably retained the strength of their magnetic fields. Among them, areas near Sedona, Arizona, and Lourdes, France, are destinations to which countless persons travel annually to experience feelings of well-being and to seek healing.

Much research and interest is now directed toward the electrical nature of life. Scientists have established beyond any doubt that all living cells are electrical in nature. The functioning of the cells and nervous system of every living being is based on direct current (DC) and pulsed DC energy. Without this energy, there is no life. Each individual cell possesses a positive electrical charge at its nucleus and a negative electrical charge on its outer membrane.

This positive-negative polarization allows each cell to function in an orderly and healthy manner. As cells perform their normal bodily functions, this electromagnetic charge wears down. The body attempts to revitalize these "tired" cells by sending pulses of electromagnetic energy from the brain through the nervous system to recharge the cells and strengthen the polarized field.

This energy can be diminished or blocked by conditions found throughout today's environment, resulting in a host of modern maladies. These range from headaches and fatigue to tumors and disruption of both circulatory and digestive systems, along with other specific and nonspecific ailments.

Noted researchers, including the U.S. Surgeon General, warn of the harmful effects of the "electric smog" from televisions, radio, radar, electric blankets, waterbed heaters, household appliances, power lines and other sources.

Sensitive instruments show that man's mushrooming alternating current (AC) electronic technology is creating interference with the earth's natural magnetic fields. Within a typical home or work environment, the AC radiation is sufficiently prolific to overpower the earth's natural magnetic field by up to 16 times. In today's buildings, the iron and steel alone can deplete the magnetic field by more than half.

The earth produces its own direct current (DC) magnetic pulses that support the natural biorhythms of all living things. However, as mentioned previously, scientists are becoming increasingly alarmed that the present-day magnetic field of the earth has and continues to diminish significantly.

A radiation researcher at Arizona State University believes that ordinary 60-cycle household AC electricity and higher frequencies such as those from radio broadcasts and radar can cause memory loss, headaches, changes in heart rate and blood chemistry and general malaise.

European scientists report such daily exposure is cumulative and contributes to sluggishness, headaches, and both digestive and circulatory problems. At the University of Colorado in Boulder, Dr. Nancy Wertheimer has reported increased cancer among children in "high current" dwellings.

According to Dr. William Adey, an American cancer researcher, this "electronic smog" can block the brain's electromagnetic signals to the cells, thereby undermining the body's disease-fighting ability and promoting tumors.

Dr. Robert O. Becker, M.D., one of America's pioneers in the field of research on regeneration and electrical currents in living things, has achieved what have been termed "miraculous" results in healing with biomagnetic therapy. He has gone so far as to speculate that electropollution, in addition to causing some cancers, may be contributing to the onslaught of such maladies as Reye's syndrome, Lyme disease, Legionnaire's disease, and AIDS.

Kyoichi Nakagawa, M.D., one of the world's foremost authorities on magnetism and its therapeutic effects on the human body, claims that the continuing degrading of earth's magnetic field, combined with man's electronic environment, is responsible for a broad range of ailments which he labels as the Magnetic Deficiency Syndrome. These ailments include stiffness of the shoulders, back, and neck, uncertain low back pain, chest pains for no specific reason, habitual headache and heaviness of the head, dizziness and insomnia for uncertain reasons, habitual constipation and general fatigue.

How Magnetic Fields Affect The Body

Another scientist whose comprehensive studies of magnetic fields and healing have been widely published is Physicist/Psychologist Dr. Buryl Payne, inventor of the first biofeedback instruments and former professor at Boston University and Goddard College. His recent books, *The Body Magnetic* and *Getting Started in Magnetic Healing* have served as authoritative handbooks for professionals and lay people alike.

According to Dr. Payne, sensitive research instruments have allowed scientists to document some of the ways magnetic fields affect living organisms. He cites specific factors now known to be involved in magnetic healing. Among them are:

• Increased blood flow with resultant increased oxygen-carrying capacity, both of which are basic to helping the body heal itself;

• Changes in migration of calcium ions which can either bring calcium ions to heal a broken bone in half the usual time, or can help move calcium away from painful, arthritic joints;

• The pH balance (acid/alkaline) of various body fluids (often out of balance in conjunction with illness or abnormal conditions) can apparently be altered by magnetic fields;

- Hormone production from the endocrine glands can be either increased or decreased by magnetic stimulation;
- Altering of enzyme activity and other biochemical processes.

As an example of specific effects created when a magnetic field is applied to the body, below are typical changes that have been documented:

- Electricity is generated in blood vessels;
- Ionized particles increase in the blood;
- Autonomic nerves are excited;
- Circulation is improved.

To better understand the implications of providing the body with an adequate magnetic environment, it is important to understand the basic movement of certain body fluids and their role in health and disease.

In a somewhat simplified explanation, as the heart pumps approximately 80 times per minute, blood in the arteries forces nutrient-laden liquid through pores in the capillaries into the cell area to nourish the cells. (This liquid is called plasma while it is in the bloodstream and is re-named "lymph" once it leaves the bloodstream.)

The blood proteins in the vessels have a high affinity for water, and aid in pulling liquid back into the blood vessels. Through the venous system, the "used" blood is returned to the heart and lungs for purification and recharging.

Because each individual cell, and the body as a whole, is an electrical generator, the cells must have oxygen to convert glucose into energy, and the balance of potassium/sodium within each cell must remain correct to keep the generators going.

The blood plasma contains numerous cells and protein molecules suspended in it. Under ordinary conditions, the normal blood pressure causes some of the blood proteins to continually seep through the tiny capillary pores into the spaces around the cells. There is not enough pressure in the cells to push these proteins back through the pores, so they must be continually removed and returned to the blood stream via the lymphatic system.

Pain and disease begin when conditions cause the capillary pores to dilate and allow the escape of significant quantities of blood proteins into the cellular area. This crowding of the proteins attracts fluid (inflammation), causes pain, and deprives some of the cells in the area of proper oxygen and nutrients, resulting in poor cellular functioning. These malfunctioning cells, if not carried away and disposed of by the lymphatic system, begin to destroy healthy cells and may keep proliferating into cancer or reenter the bloodstream and cause leukemia.

If the lymphatic system completely fails to function and these blood proteins become trapped throughout the body, death can occur within hours.

According to Dr. C. Samuel West, chemist and internationally recognized lymphologist, trapped blood proteins are the one common denominator present in all pain and disease...

In citing circumstances which can cause trapped blood proteins, Dr. West lists the following: shallow breathing, improper exercise, shock, stress, anger, fear, tea, coffee, liquor, tobacco, drugs, salt, sugar, fat, high-cholesterol food, too much meat and others.

Many years of research and clinical application have shown that the simple introduction of a magnetic field can provide stimulation and enhancement of the lymphatic system, as well as every cell within the body. The magnetic field does not heal; it merely aids the cells in creating an optimum environment in which the body can begin to heal itself. Between the circulatory, lymphatic and neurological effects, outstanding advances in health can be obtained.

Many biomagnetic practitioners are now offering education, treatment, and magnetic devices to those seeking alternative health care. Among the most viable of these options is a magnetic sleep system developed in Japan. Users are able to sleep nightly within a cocoon of balanced magnetic energy to revitalize their bodies, with the system providing ongoing effectiveness levels. Manufacturers of these magnetotherapeutic mattresses are claiming that the use of their products replaces the magnetism lost through natural decay, interference caused by electromagnetic fields and metallic structures in our environments.

Clinical Test of Magnetic Mattresspads
By Dr. Kazuo Shimodaira

The mattresspads used in this study were typical full-size pads containing 124 permanent ferrite magnets with magnetic field strengths of 750-950 gauss each. The pads themselves were made of two sheets of felt with the magnets sandwiched between them. The felt sheets were then wrapped in a cloth cover. The total number of subjects of this double-blind clinical experiment was 431 (216 male, 215 female). 375 subjects were given the magnetic pads, 56 were given nonmagnetic pads. None of the 431 subjects knew which pad they were sleeping on. Subjects selected for the experiment were those with chief complaints related to: neck and shoulder pain, back and lower back pain, back pain (general), lower limb pain, insomnia, fatigue.

To determine the presence of any side effects, blood pressure, hemoglobin, number of erythrocytes, and number of leukocytes were examined before and after the use of the mattresspads. Besides blood sedimentation, TP, COL, ALP, GOY, GPT, Na, and K were also examined, as were functions of the kidneys, liver, pancreas, and the entire circulatory system.

Results

Symptom	Cases	Positive Results	%	No Results	%
Neck and shoulder pain	66	47	71.2	19	28.8
Back and lower back pain	76	61	80.3	15	19.7
Back pain (general)	31	25	80.7	6	19.3
Lower limb pain	68	54	79.4	14	20.6
Insomnia	70	61	87.1	9	12.9
Fatigue	64	53	82.8	11	17.2

Out of 375 total subjects with symptoms, 301 (80.27%) reported positive results. 74 cases (19.73%) reported no results.

Time of Response

The percentage of subjects who realized the effect of the magnetic mattresspad within 3 days:

Neck and shoulder pain	46.9%
Back and lower back pain	50.0%
Back pain	38.7%
Lower limb pain	54.4%
Insomnia	64.3%
Fatigue	57.8%

Out of 375 total subjects who slept on the magnetic mattresspads, 200 (53.3%) realized the effects within 3 days. Over 70% realized the effects within 5 days.

Testing for side effects was conducted at the conclusion of the experiment. Symptoms such as tinnitus, headache, hearing problems, visual disturbances, vertigo, palpitation, perceptive abnormality, motorial disturbance, fever, digestive disturbance, cutaneous symptoms, and other clinical symptoms to suggest any side effects were found to be totally absent. Extensive testing was also done before and after the experiment to check functions of kidney, liver, pancreas, blood pressure, and the circulatory system. No clinical symptoms were found to indicate any side effects whatsoever.

Conclusion

Dr. Shimodaira's conclusions of this yearlong study conducted in three of Japan's foremost hospitals: "The magnetized health mattresspad is proven to be effective on neck and shoulder pain, back and lower back pain, lower limb pain, insomnia, and fatigue, and to have no side effects."

References

Bansal, Dr. H.L., *Magnet Therapy*

Bansal, Dr. H.L., and Bansal, Dr. R.S., *Magnetic Cure for Common Diseases*

Becker, Robert O., MD, *Cross Currents*

Becker, Robert O., MD, & Selden, Gary, *The Body Electric*

Breakthrough Media, Inc., *Magnetic Devices for Self Use*

Brennan, Barbara Ann, *Hands of Light*

Brennan, Barbara Ann, *Light Emerging*

Callahan, Phillip S., *Ancient Mysteries, Modern Visions*

Cerney, J. V., *Acupuncture Without Needles*

Davis, Albert Roy, & Rawls, Walter C., Jr., *Magnetism and Its Effects on The Living System*

Davis, Albert Roy, & Rawls, Walter C., Jr., *The Magnetic Effect*

Davis, Albert Roy, & Rawls, Walter C., Jr., *The Rainbow In Your Hands*

Hacmac, Edward A., DC, *An Overview of Biomagnetic Therapeutics*

Hannemann, Holger, *Magnet Therapy: Balancing Your Body's Energy Flow for Self-Healing*, Sterling Publishing Company, 387 Park Avenue South, New York, NY, 10016

Kervran, C. L., *Biological Transmutation*

O'Brien, Jim, Revolutionary New Magnetic Therapy KO's Arthritis Pain, *Your Health*, April 6, 1993

Payne, Dr. Buryl, *The Body Magnetic*

Payne, Dr. Buryl, *Getting Started in Magnetic Healing*

Suplee, Curt, Magnetism—The Force That's Always With You, *The Washington Post*, Page H1, December 14, 1994

References from *Why Magnetic Field Therapy Works*,
by Leane E. Roffey

1. Upledger, John E., and Vredevoogd, Jon D., "Craniosacral Therapy," Eastland Press, Seattle, WA, c. 1983.
2. Shea, Michael J., "A Manual for Cranial Mobilization Technique," Shea Educational Group, Juno Beach, FL, c. 1992.
3. Moe, Bruce, Giddings, John A., Cosby, Richard S., "Electrophysiology," Measurements & Data Corporation, 2994 W. Liberty Ave., Pittsburgh, PA, c. 1981.
4. Ilmonlemi, Risto J., "Neuromagnetic Measurements with a 24-Channel SQUID Magnetometer," Annual International Conference of the IEEE Engineering in Medicine and Biology Society, Vol. 12, No. 3, 1990.
5. R. Hari, H. Hamalainen, M. Hamalainen, J. Kekoni, M. Sams, and J. Tiihonen, "Separate finger representations at the human second somalosensory cortex," *Neuroscience*, in press (1990).
6. Kirschvink, Joseph L., Kobayashi, Atsuko, and Woodford, Barbara J., "Magnetite Biomineralization in the Human Brain," Division of Geological & Planetary Science, The California Institute of Technology, Pasadena, CA.
7. Nakagawa, Kyoichi, "Magnetic Field Deficiency Syndrome and Magnetic Treatment," Translation of the article which appeared in the Japan Medical Journal, No. 274S, Dec. 4, 1976.
8. Lapedes, Daniel N., editor-in-chief, "McGraw Hill Dictionary of Physics and Mathematics," c. 1978.
9. Oschman, James L., "Structure and Properties of Ground Substances," Amer. Zool., 24:199-215 (1984).
10. Oschman, James L., "The Connective Tissue and Myofascial Systems," The Rolf Institute, c. 1987.

To order products
or to
obtain information about
Magnetic Field Therapy
contact:

Inner Search
Foundation, Inc.

P.O. Box 10382
McLean, Virginia 22102

or call

703-448-3362

 INNER SEARCH FOUNDATION, INC.
McLean, Virginia

To order additional copies call:

Inner Search Foundation, Inc.

703-448-3362

Quantity Discount

Price for: 1 - 5 $9.95
                6 - 15 $8.95
                16 - 49 $7.95
                50+ $7.00

Plus $5.00 for UPS Ground or
$8.00 for FED-EX Economy.
Call for shipping quote on 30+.

Send check or money order to:

Inner Search Foundation, Inc.
P.O. Box 10382
McLean, VA 22102-1502

For a complete listing of products, request
a catalogue when ordering.